Human Well-Being Research and Policy Making

Series Editors

Richard J. Estes, School of Social Policy & Practice, University of Pennsylvania, Philadelphia, PA, USA

M. Joseph Sirgy, Department of Marketing, Virginia Polytechnic Institute & State University, Blacksburg, VA, USA

This series creates a dialogue between well-being scholars and well-being public policy makers.

Well-being theory, research and practice are essentially interdisciplinary in nature and embrace contributions from all disciplines within the social sciences. With the exception of leading economists, the policy relevant contributions of social scientists are widely scattered and lack the coherence and integration needed to more effectively inform the actions of policy makers.

Contributions in the series focus on one more of the following four aspects of well-being and public policy:

- Discussions of the public policy and well-being focused on particular nations and worldwide regions
- Discussions of the public policy and well-being in specialized sectors of policy making such as health, education, work, social welfare, housing, transportation, use of leisure time
- Discussions of public policy and well-being associated with particular population groups such as women, children and youth, the aged, persons with disabilities and vulnerable populations
- Special topics in well-being and public policy such as technology and well-being, terrorism and well-being, infrastructure and well-being.

More information about this series at http://www.springer.com/series/15692

Vijay Kumar Shrotryia

Human Well-Being
and Policy in South Asia

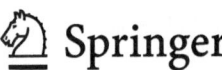 Springer

Vijay Kumar Shrotryia
Department of Commerce
University of Delhi
Delhi, India

ISSN 2522-5367   ISSN 2522-5375 (electronic)
Human Well-Being Research and Policy Making
ISBN 978-3-030-33269-3   ISBN 978-3-030-33270-9 (eBook)
https://doi.org/10.1007/978-3-030-33270-9

This Springer imprint is published by the registered company Springer Nature Switzerland AG
The registered company address is: Gewerbestrasse 11, 6330 Cham, Switzerland

For my parents
Sri B. P. Shrotryia (late)
and Smt. Sharda Devi

Preface

Bhutan has played a key role in introducing the concept of happiness and well-being to me and to the world as well. I worked there between 1993 and 2002 and developed an academic interest in the study of quality of life, happiness and well-being. The emphasis on policies towards improving quality of life and well-being through the focus on Gross National Happiness rather than gross domestic product has been a pivotal development. It has been able to generate academic interest among social scientists and policymakers. Bhutan is one of the smallest countries in South Asia, containing less than a million people in total population. Though it is one of the least developed nations across globe, its primary focus has not been to develop economically; rather it has been to prioritize happiness over income. This development philosophy has made Bhutan unique and noble.

Generally, human beings aspire to be happy. State policy works to facilitate this human aspiration. The policies are crafted to create, maintain and harness those conditions which are conducive to assure human well-being. The previous century witnessed significant transformations with respect to the development of physical infrastructure amid geopolitical changes, turmoil and adjustments. New economic systems to measure social and human progress were introduced which gained universal acceptance by development institutions and the developed nations of the world. However, overemphasis on economic policies and growth, leading towards increase in income, did not positively translate in improving human well-being vis-à-vis human happiness. The same is true of South Asia. South Asia has eight sovereign countries, each with diversities in religion, language and culture. It is the most populous and the most densely populated region in the world and possesses rich resources with potential to become one of the most vibrant economic regions of the world in general. This book is designed to shift policy focus towards improving the general well-being of people in this region.

A couple of years ago, I had written a chapter titled "History of Well-Being in South Asia" (co-author Krishna Mazumdar) for *The Pursuit of Human Well-Being—The Untold Global History*, edited by Professor Richard J. Estes and Professor M. Joseph Sirgy. While preparing that chapter, we realized that it could be expanded into a book of this kind. The motivation, guidance and academic mentoring by both of the editors culminated into this book. This book is organized around policies in all the eight South Asian countries (Afghanistan, Bangladesh, Bhutan, India, the Maldives, Nepal, Pakistan and Sri Lanka), specifically focusing on policy relating to education, health, governance and economic development. It discusses vulnerabilities related to these broad themes with the support of data published by the World Bank and other agencies. It then identifies and compares the indicators related to these domains in order to make appropriate recommendations.

This book is divided into five chapters, which include the "An Introduction to Human Well-Being, Policy and South Asia Region", "Human Well-Being Indicators in South Asia Region", "Major Policy Interventions for Human Well-Being in South Asia", "Human Well-Being Policy and Discussion" and "Conclusion and the Way Forward". I have incorporated a brief discussion on Bhutan's journey to adopt the Gross National Happiness metric in order to provide background information, practical aspects and outcome as obtained from the published reports and statistics, and have discussed the contributions made by some pathbreakers (Mohd. Yunus from Bangladesh, Mehbub Ul Haque and Malala Yousafzai from Pakistan, and Kailash Satyarthi from India) from the region in the recent past wherever relevant. The book concludes with a summary of the outcomes and a note on building a case for considering human well-being as a future policy focus apart from GDP. It outlines expected policy interventions and finally provides a summary of the strengths, weaknesses, opportunities, and threats of each of the countries in the region.

It is my hope that this book will help scholars gain a better understanding and perspective of the region and will guide policymakers towards appropriate policy frameworks for each of these countries, leading towards improved quality of life, vis-à-vis human well-being. I also hope that the information provided will help the reader articulate an alternative to GDP-driven policies and help reduce the class gap through a sustainable policy framework.

Delhi, India   Vijay Kumar Shrotryia

Acknowledgements

This book would not have been initiated without motivation from Prof. Richard J. Estes (University of Pennsylvania) and Prof. M. J. Sirgy (Virginia Polytechnic Institute and State University) who persistently reposed their confidence in me for taking up the project. As series editors, they have helped immensely in shaping this book through their guidance, observations and comments during the journey. I would like to thank them profusely for all their support and bearing with me for going beyond the committed deadlines.

The unceasing support of my doctoral students (members of the HappLab) made my task relatively easier. I am grateful to Shashank for digging into background data from different sources, Reema for converting tables into figures, and Upasana for compiling the details of profiles of people and projects from South Asia. Thanks are also due to the Geographic Information Officer, under Geospatial Information Section of the United Nations who provided timely permission to use the political map of South Asia in this book.

Prashanth Ravichandran from Springer deserves thanks for driving me to complete the manuscript in a timely manner. Sudarshan Khanna came to my rescue for copy editing, and completed the job despite having health problems. I would like to thank him for his committed efforts and humility.

I wish to thank my wife, Ragini, and daughter, Akshada, for being strong pillars of strength. They have been a source of constant inspiration throughout.

Acknowledgements

Contents

About the Author

Dr. Vijay Kumar Shrotryia is Professor in the Department of Commerce, Delhi School of Economics, University of Delhi, India. He has taught in Bhutan for around a decade and developed an interest in the study of quality of life, happiness and Gross National Happiness. He did a UNFPA-funded project on studying the quality of life of local village/town-area residents while in Bhutan and conducted two follow-up surveys after leaving Bhutan. He co-authored a chapter titled "History of Human Well-Being in South Asia" for a volume (*The Pursuit of Human Well-Being—The Untold Global History*) edited by Dr. Richard Estes and Dr. Joe Sirgy and published by Springer. His academic interest includes study of well-being, happiness, satisfaction and corporate strategies. He has recently completed a monograph titled *In Defense of Inclusion of Happiness in Public Policy for India* for the India Policy Foundation, New Delhi. He is involved in the activities of Rajya Anand Sansthan (State Happiness Institute), Madhya Pradesh (India), as an expert.

Abbreviations

AFG	Afghanistan
ALR	Adult Literacy Rate
ASHA	Accredited Social Health Activist
AYUSH	Ayurveda, Yoga and Naturopathy, Unani, Siddha and Homoeopathy
BAN	Bangladesh
BHU	Bhutan
BRAC	Bangladesh Rural Advancement Committee
CIAA	Commission for the Investigation of Abuse of Authority
CSR	Corporate Social Responsibility
DNT	Druk Nyamrup Tshogpa
DPT	Druk Phuensum Tshogpa
EAS	East Asia and Pacific
ECCD	Early Childhood Care and Development
ECS	Europe and Central Asia
EFA	Education For All
EMU	Euro Area
FDI	Foreign Direct Investment
FYP	Five-Year Plans
GDP	Gross Domestic Product
GFHR	Global Forum for Health Research
GNH	Gross National Happiness
GNHC	Gross National Happiness Commission
GST	Goods and Services Tax
GWP	Gallup World Poll
HDI	Human Development Index
HDR	Human Development Report
HPI	Happy Planet Index
HWB	Human Well-Being
ICT	Information and Computer Technology
ILO	International Labour Organization

IMR	Infant Mortality Rate
INR	Indian Rupee
IPCC	Intergovernmental Panel on Climate Change
KRA	Key Result Area
LCN	Latin America and Caribbean
LLC	Limited Liability Companies
MAL	The Maldives
MDG	Millennium Development Goals
MMR	Maternal Mortality Rate
MNREGA	Mahatma Gandhi National Rural Employment Guarantee Act
MPI	Multidimensional Poverty Index
NCP	Nepali Congress Party
NEF	New Economics Foundation
NEP	Nepal
NFE	Non-Formal Education
NGO	Non-Governmental Organization
NHM	National Health Mission
NHRC	National Human Rights Commission
NPI	National Prosperity Index
NRHM	National Rural Health Mission
NUHM	National Urban Health Mission
OECD	Organization for Economic Co-operation and Development
OPHI	Oxford Poverty and Human Development Initiative
PAK	Pakistan
PPP	Purchasing Power Parity
PURA	Providing Urban amenities in Rural Areas
QOL	Quality of Life
RGOB	Royal Government of Bhutan
RTE	Right to Education
RTI	Right to Information
RUSA	Rashtriya Uchchatar Shiksha Abhiyan
SA	South Asia
SAARC	South Asian Association for Regional Cooperation
SAFTA	South Asia Free Trade Agreement
SAPTA	South Asia Preferential Trade Agreement
SDG	Sustainable Development Goal
SEHAT	System Enhancement for Health Action in Transition
SEN	Special Education Needs
SLK	Sri Lanka
SLTHP	Second Long-Term Health Plan
SSA	Sarva Shiksha Abhiyan
SSF	Sub-Saharan Africa
STEM	Science, Technology, Engineering, and Mathematics
SWB	Subjective Well-Being
TT2	Tetanus Toxoid

UK	United Kingdom
UN	United Nations
UNDP	United Nations Development Programme
UNESCO	United Nations Educational, Scientific and Cultural Organization
US	United States
USAID	United States Agency for International Development
USD	United States Dollar
USSR	Union of Soviet Socialist Republics
WDH	World Database of Happiness
WHO	World Health Organization
WHR	World Happiness Report
WTO	World Trade Organization
WVS	World Values Survey

List of Figures

List of Tables

List of Tables

List of Boxes

List of Boxes

Chapter 1
An Introduction to Human Well-Being, Policy and South Asia Region

I often ask myself what is the purpose of our lives and I conclude that life's purpose is to be happy. We have no guarantee what will happen in the future, but we live in hope. That's what keeps us going.
[Dalai Lama][a]

Abstract This chapter highlights the importance of human well-being (HWB) in general and in South Asia more particularly, taking its direction from South Asia's emphasis on religious beliefs and the region's very rich cultural history that has shaped human civilizations worldwide. A link between human development and HWB is established in order to argue the importance of public policy in improving living conditions for eight of the region's largest and most influential countries, now and in the past, e.g., Afghanistan, Bangladesh, Bhutan, India, the Maldives, Nepal, Pakistan, and Sri Lanka. Brief histories of these countries are given, which demonstrate contemporary developments in their socio-economic sphere. The geographic size and demographics of these eight countries and the region as a whole is depicted for policy consideration. The emergence of South Asian Association for Regional Cooperation (SAARC) as a unifying agency for all South Asian countries to pursue common goals, has been described in the chapter. Towards the end of the chapter, synopses of the other chapters are provided.

Keywords Human well-being · South Asia · Public policy · Afghanistan · Bangladesh · Bhutan · India · The Maldives · Nepal · Pakistan · Sri Lanka

1.1 Introduction

The quintessential public policy of a state is aimed towards facilitating human well-being (HWB) for all its citizens and to ensure that they lead their lives secured, peaceful, and in the peak of health with a sense of dignity. Public programs—often in the form of multi-year strategic plans—in cooperation with nongovernmental

---

[a]His Holiness Dalai Lama posted this tweet on May 7, 2018. Accessed from https://twitter.com/DalaiLama/status/993422714646941696.

© Springer Nature Switzerland AG 2020
V. K. Shrotryia, *Human Well-Being and Policy in South Asia*, Human Well-Being Research and Policy Making, https://doi.org/10.1007/978-3-030-33270-9_1

organizations, assign priority to areas of special need and identify those sectors which need special attention through policies that can be implemented. This process as taken up by the state, also includes earmarking allocations and subsequent effective delivery for the cause of common well-being of inhabitants and beneficiaries. The role of the state becomes more important in those countries that are striving to achieve greater social and economic progress. South Asia is one such group of countries. Though the index of economic progress in this region has improved gradually, progress on all fronts still needs acceleration to achieve new heights.

It is in this light that this volume is organized to analyze the region from the perspective of well-being and the state in all eight South Asian countries and to articulate the policy initiatives and their effects on the HWB through social, economic, and development indicators. Secondary data published in annual analytical and statistical reports (World Bank reports, World Development reports, Human Development reports etc.) are used to bring some plausible conclusions for guiding future policy in the required direction.

1.2   Importance of Human Well-Being

The ultimate goal of human life is assumed to be the achievement and maintenance of human well-being. It is a universal belief that humans want to lead peaceful and happy lives. Different religions view this ultimate goal in different ways, though in the end—in an abstract form—the goal remains same. While Christianity focuses on establishing a Kingdom of God by destroying evil forces, Hinduism considers *Ram-Rajya* as an ideal state where all citizens live in peace and harmony. Islam views life as being meaningful and fulfilling by submitting to *Allah* and to His Will (as interpreted and understood by individual members and their clerics). In the same way, other religions also preach and practice to make life meaningful vis-à-vis improving human life conditions. Religion guides efforts, provides larger vision, and paves the way towards encouraging believers to serve humanity.

The academic study of well-being[1] has remained a domain of economists, psychologists, sociologists, and political scientists, depending on their own expertise. In subjective terms, well-being is viewed as evaluation of an individual's life situation or 'state.' This construct has been broadly described through different expressions such as welfare, quality of life, life satisfaction, standard of living, and happiness. It is two dimensional, namely hedonic and eudaiemonic. Both are complementary in nature.

Human development, over a period of time, has also emerged as one of the related fields for assessment and policy focus. Largely these overlapping terms address issues related to HWB and, in one way or the other, reflect on its intent to improve

---

[1] For detailed discussion see Gasper (2004).

living conditions resulting in well-meaning, peaceful, and happy lives. Absence of suffering coupled with good health, fulfilling basic needs, and having concern for humanity at large is part of HWB. The focus of all human efforts is to attain these goals, and efforts are to be made at all levels to realize them—individual, national, and global. Ideally, we all wish to live in healthy, harmonious, happy, and peaceful world. At the individual level, the primary goal is to be able to fulfill basic needs and to grow into a being with freedom to choose. People must have the means to earn a living to satisfy their needs and beyond. Their accumulated resources and effort to improve their living conditions culminates into satisfaction with life overall.

The state, nation, or government has primary responsibility of caring for its citizens by establishing the rule of law to govern effectively, to formulate effective public policy, and to make provisions for basic necessities. Governance should be transparent, sustaining, and effective. The purpose of public policy is to assure well-being by fulfilling the needs of citizens and encouraging the development of an ecosystem promoting freedom and conditions in which choices can be exercised. Provisions of good healthcare and education helps people improve their lives as they are able to take care of their health and capitalize on available opportunities through appropriate employment and/or entrepreneurship. Access to education, healthcare, and social welfare services with effective mechanisms under conditions of freedom and choice help improve social well-being, promoting competence and increased individual capabilities. This has been the basic premise of human development. The whole idea of human development has been to allow people the ability to broaden their repertoire of choices that can improve their general well-being.

Apart from public policy, the South Asian countries also invest in building better relationships with other nations so that they are able to learn from each other and share resources for improving living conditions. Economic policies are formulated to eventually affect household income, which ideally results in economic empowerment and wealthier nations. Such creation of wealth (and its justified distribution) improves HWB and possibly makes the nation state self-sufficient. As such, HWB is viewed as a multidimensional construct having physical, psychological, economic, and social well-being dimensions.

Globally, responsible international agencies spend a great deal of resources in order to eliminate food deficiency, which is a precondition to make the world healthy, happy, and peaceful. 'Education for all' and 'health for all' are common goals of philanthropies across globe, including that of the World Bank. It is expected that these common goals improve physical as well as mental (and psychological) well-being of citizens. This shall extend equal opportunities to the citizens to explore and find the purpose of human life. It would also lead and direct their efforts with renewed concentration. Ideally, it should also augment their attitude towards life. The main aim of human life is to serve others, express sympathy sensibly and act in such a way that displays the resolve for helping others, minus sense of greediness. Ancient Vedic philosophy appropriately vouches for four objectives (in order) for the fulfillment of the purpose of human life, viz., *Dharma* (righteousness), *Arth* (wealth), *Kama* (controlled fulfillment of desire), and *Moksha* (salvation). This philosophy reflects a broader perspective of HWB by acknowledging the importance of all human needs and aspirations. The same philosophy guides human efforts for achieving them and provides a framework for public policy as well.

The present work concentrates on the South Asian region comprising eight nations[2] which are more or less at a similar level of economic development, though varying in terms of human development at large. The nation states of South Asia are passing through difficult times as inequalities are on the rise and internal problems are consuming much of their resources. These conditions pose a much greater challenge for policymakers to prioritize resource allocation.

1.3   Role of Public Policy in Improving Human Well-Being

The framing of policies gets inspired through the intent of visualizing positive and happy world and its conditions that support the cause of human existence whether it is to meet basic individual and social needs or global well-being. A state puts effort to draft, design and implement policies so that human life conditions are improved and quality of life is assured. Such a direction for all public policies becomes important for economically poor or/and nations in the developing process. Chakrabarti and Sanyal (2017) stated that:

> Public policy is a matter of life and death – of people, societies, even the entire world. It determines the quality of ordinary citizens' lives, the prosperity of nations, peace, security, and sustainability at a geo-political level. It makes the difference between breakout nations and failed states. ... Equally critical is the most complex and challenging task of implementing it, negotiating a vexing maze of organizational psychology and human systems in a fast-changing environment. (p. xiv)

Hence, public policy has a close link with the quality of life enjoyed by citizens and their well-being. The whole exercise of developing public policy becomes futile if it becomes ineffective, or if not implemented sensibly despite being effective. Ineffective public policy amounts to human ill-being. Three steps are important in developing public policy: policy formulation, implementation, and evaluation. Any policy framed for the welfare of common public of a state should be considered as public policy be it providing quality education at all levels, better health facilities, maintenance of law and order by enacting good governance and anti-corruption measures, protecting environment, developing poverty alleviation programs, and similar initiatives.

These are central issues to be made part of any public policy designing process across globe. However, these issues are more relevant for the South Asian countries as the region is still currently developing and conditions of living or well-being

---

[2]Official names of these eight nations in alphabetical order are: Afghanistan—The Islamic Republic of Afghanistan; Bangladesh—The People's Republic of Bangladesh; Bhutan—The Kingdom of Bhutan (or *Druk Yul*); India—The Republic of India; the Maldives—Republic of Maldives; Nepal—The Federal Democratic Republic of Nepal; Pakistan—The Islamic Republic of Pakistan; Sri Lanka—The Democratic Socialist Republic of Sri Lanka.

are much lower than the world average.[3] Across the globe, innovation and development in technology has transformed lives of people, and South Asia is no exception. The implementation and monitoring of public policy initiatives are made efficient and timely through effective use of technology. Hence, investment in building technological infrastructure becomes a priority for a state. In the modern world, policy analysis and evaluation are assisted by technology, and real time data is generated for effective decision-making, which contributes to efficient public policy monitoring.

Policy outcomes are measured and reflected through the data from social indicators. For developing economies, as that of the countries in South Asian region, it befits all the more, as the prevailing situation demands better concentration on the concerning issues in public policy. It is in this context that the present work is being organized to reflect on the status of quality of life vis-à-vis HWB, across nations of the South Asian region and to analyze public policy interventions and their subsequent outcomes. Further it is aimed at providing major guideline framework for future policy making.

1.4   South Asia Region: An Introduction

The history of the region, its geographic and political landscape, determines its policy focus calling for improvement in human life conditions. The region enjoys rich cultural heritage providing base for concern for HWB. It has valuable reservoirs of natural capital and is bestowed with all weather conditions. Though the region has been mostly democratic, it has faced many political challenges which have had a greater influence on the region's public policy. This section provides a brief background concerning demography, geography, and history of the region for better understanding of its people, problems and prospects.

South Asia region, as used in this text, follows the World Bank composition which is widely accepted. It consists of eight sovereign nations (Fig. 1.1) including Afghanistan, Bangladesh, Bhutan, the Maldives, Nepal, India, Pakistan, and Sri Lanka. It is geographically situated in the southern extremity of the Eurasian continent. Importantly among the top ten most populated nations of the world, South Asia has three of them, namely India, Pakistan, and Bangladesh. As around 75% of population (and 62% of land area) (Fig. 1.3) of this region resides in India, it is also called the 'Indian Subcontinent'.[4] "The terms 'South Asia' and 'India' refer, in the first instance, to a vast geographical space stretching from the Himalayan mountain ranges in the north to the Indian Ocean in the south; and from the valley of the Indus in the west to the plains of the Brahmaputra in the east" (Bose & Jalal, 2004, p. 3).

---

[3]The chapter by Estes and Sirgy (2017) discusses the trends in well-being across globe with the help of secondary data, more specifically between 1980 and 2013.

[4]Mohammad-Arif (2014) has articulated the use of the term 'South Asia' and 'Indian subcontinent' in detail covering need of an identity (area studies in American universities) and theoretical perspectives on the phraseology and popular use of the term for identity, representation and convenience.

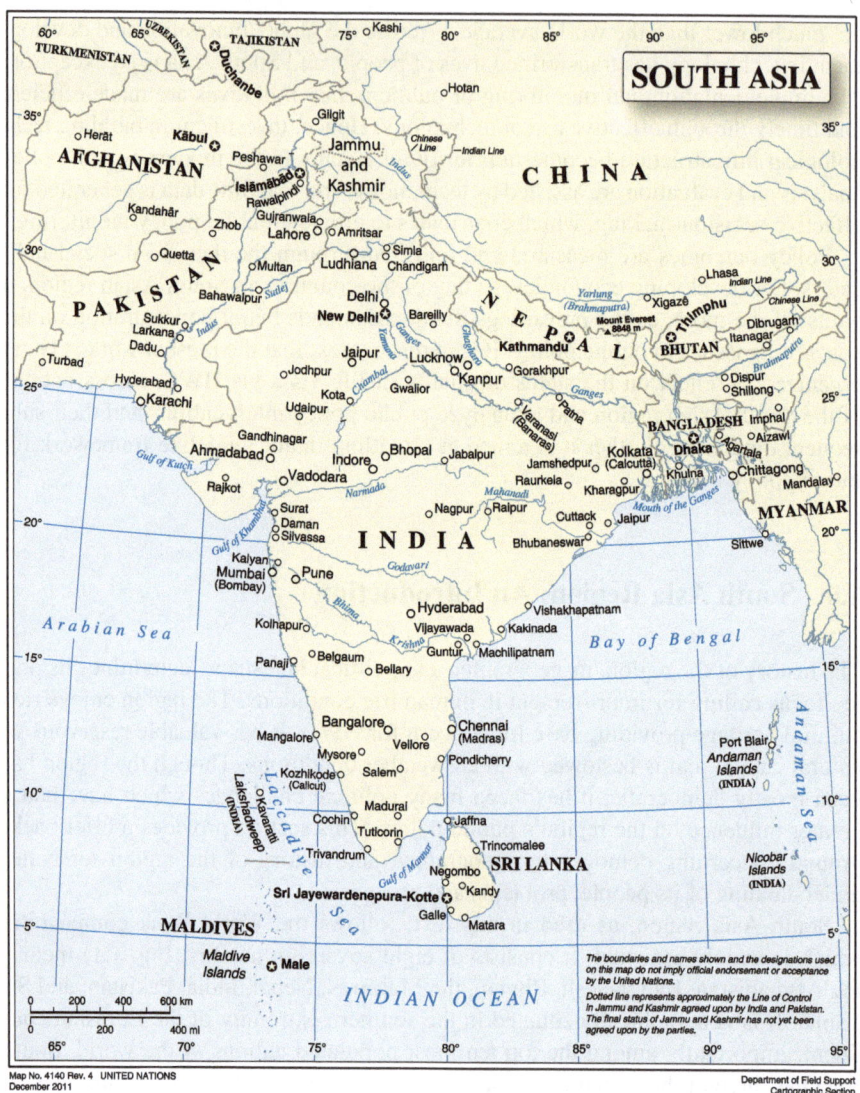

Fig. 1.1 Political map of South Asia

Around one-fourth of the population of the world lives in this region; though this is only roughly 4% of world's land mass (Table 1.1, Fig. 1.2), which makes it the most densely populated geographic region on the planet. It is also considered to be the most culturally diverse region (Petraglia & Boivin, 2014, p. 339) as some of the key religions of the world such as Hinduism, Buddhism, Jainism and Sikhism have originated here. This region houses the world's largest population of Hindus, Jains, and Sikhs. Most of the residents of this region are Hindus (67%); Muslim (31%);

Table 1.1 Land area and population composition in South Asian Region

Countries	Land Area			Population		
	In '000 square km	Share in South Asia (%)	Share in world (%)	In millions	Share in South Asia (%)	Share in world (%)
Afghanistan (AFG)	652.86	13.68	0.57176	35.53	1.98	0.47182
Bangladesh (BAN)	130.17	2.73	0.11410	164.67	9.21	2.18674
Bhutan (BHU)	38.12	0.80	0.03344	0.81	0.05	0.01072
India (IND)	2,973.19	62.31	2.60427	1,339.18	74.88	17.78375
Maldives (MAL)	3.00	0.01	0.00026	0.44	0.02	0.00579
Nepal (NEP)	143.35	3.00	0.12539	29.30	1.64	0.38916
Pakistan (PAK)	770.88	16.16	0.67541	197.02	11.02	2.61629
Sri Lanka (SLK)	62.71	1.31	0.05475	21.44	1.20	0.28477

Source Compiled from World Bank database as updated in September 2018

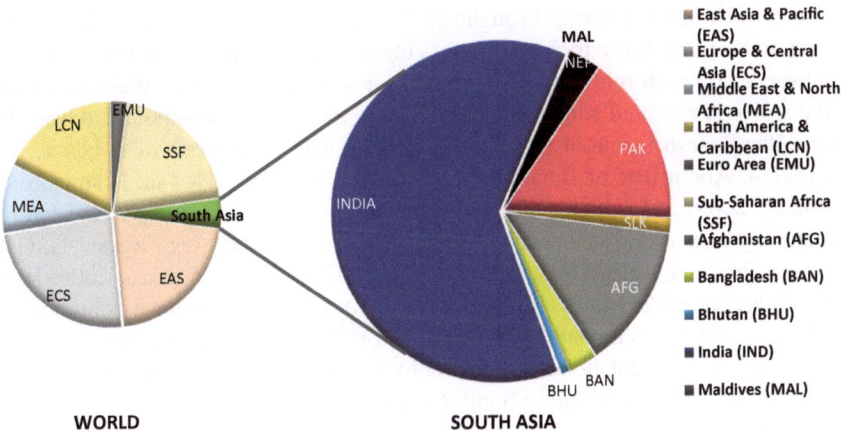

Fig. 1.2 Land area: world vis-à-vis South Asia

and the remaining are Jains, Sikhs, Buddhists and Christians. Major religions of this region are Islam (predominantly in Afghanistan, Bangladesh, the Maldives, and Pakistan), Hinduism (predominantly in India and Nepal), and Buddhism (predominantly in Bhutan and Sri Lanka).

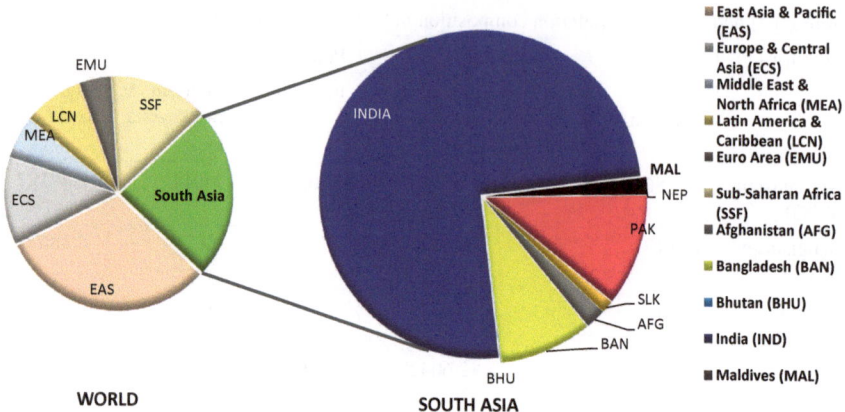

Fig. 1.3 Population: world vis-à-vis South Asia

The population density of South Asia region is the highest in the world (Table 1.1, Fig. 1.3), ranging from a high of 1454 people per km^2 for the Maldives followed by Bangladesh with 1265 people per km^2 to a low of 21 people per km^2 for Bhutan. The population density for India is 450 persons per km^2. South Asia is subject to frequent floods, mudslides, earthquakes, and extreme weather conditions, making it one of the most consistently geologically vulnerable areas in the world. Casualties and deaths associated with these natural disasters are extraordinarily high, as is the level of human suffering brought on by these frequent disasters. Though the governments have shown their seriousness towards improving the conditions of such occurrences through relevant programs for the welfare of citizens, the risks to life and property associated with these disasters, as aforesaid, get compounded over the years. Bangladesh is one of the most vulnerable nations in terms of floods across the region. About half of Bangladesh is flooded each year (Dewan, Nishigaki, & Komatsu, 2003) and is highly likely to experience complete flooding in the future, threatening its survival as a sovereign nation. Various studies (e.g., Agrawala, Ota, Ahmed, Smith, & Aalst, 2003; Dewan et al., 2003; Hofer & Messerli, 2006; Huq, 2002; Schiermeier, 2014; World Bank, 2000; etc.) on Bangladesh have examined the challenges it faces as a result of the recurrent re-building of homes and structures in response to frequent flood. "A destructive combination of earthquakes, floods, droughts and other hazards make South Asia, the world's most disaster-prone region" (Oxfam International, 2008, p. i).

Countries throughout South Asia experience high death rates, extensive property damage, and a profound sense of physical insecurity due to the harsh realities of the extreme physical environment in which they live.[5] Bhutan, through its belief in Gross National Happiness has been able to deal with disasters at an emotional level as they spiritually get prepared better to cope with disaster (Shrotryia, 2013). It does

---

[5]See Green (2012), Kumar and Narayan (2007), Raychaudhuri (1985), etc.

not mean that they do not strive to avoid and overcome it or just surrender, but when things are beyond control, their spiritual belief helps them. South Asia is helped by other nations within the region as well as other countries beyond the region, apart from the generous support of international agencies and NGOs who tackle disasters of a grievous nature and scale.

The South Asian region possesses two major characteristics: (1) Geographically, culturally, economically, philosophically, and historically, the region is Indo-centric, which means that Indian culture has, in one way or another, influenced all of the countries of the region; (2) the power structure is unbalanced and asymmetric (Muni, 1979). The geography, culture, politics and history of the region is assimilated in such a way that people from almost all religions have lived together for a long period of time. It is also evidenced that the geography of India, which houses around 75% population of the region, is vulnerable to invaders from the northwest (Kaplan, 2010). The first major civilization in South Asia was the Indus Valley Civilization, covering present day northern India, Afghanistan, and Pakistan. Pakistan and Bangladesh were part of India before the British Raj came to end in 1947 through the Indian Independence Act passed by the British Parliament in July 1947. The Indian Independence Act dictated the settlement of two dominions in India to be known respectively as India and Pakistan, with complete withdrawal of control by pre-independence India.

It was on August 14, 1947 when Pakistan was created as a Muslim nation. The Muslim League was demanding an independent state for Muslims. Mohammad Ali Jinnah along with Sir Syed Ahmed Khan advocated for the creation of a two-nation state and asked for the formation of such a state in the Lahore resolution of 1940. "Looking for a way to gather together a hopelessly scattered flock, Jinnah's resort to religion had nothing to do with his ideological convictions. This was the most practical way of mobilizing a community divided by politics but defined by religion" (Bose & Jalal, 2004, p. 146). The partition of India into two nations was the "result of a fundamental disagreement about the nature of India's civilizational nationhood" (Sanyal, 2012, p. 260).

The creation of Pakistan was marred by brutal communal clashes and the massive movement of Muslims from India to Pakistan, and Hindus and Sikhs from Pakistan to India. This displacement of more than 14 million people due solely to religious strife caused mental anguish for countless families. Scholars in literature, such as Saadat Hasan Manto, Khushwant Singh, Salman Rushdie, Amitav Ghosh, and others, have expressed the pain of partition through emotive stories and narratives across the region.[6] Though today India faces conflict with Pakistan to the west and with China to the northeast, these conflicts are very different because—historically and religiously—the ties between India and Pakistan are much closer than the ties between India and China. On one hand, the relationship between the two countries has been

---

[6]Rituparna Roy through this literary commentary on the work of authors on the partition brilliantly put forth the plight of people belonging to different strata, religion, and gender. This explains how the partition affected human lives and their well-being (see Roy, 2010).

characterized by similarities and dissimilarities in religious practices and, on the other hand, political claims on Kashmir have adversely affected their relationship.

Pakistan is world's sixth most populated country and its economy is dominated by the service sector. It shares its borders with India to the east, Afghanistan to the northwest, and Iran to the west. The Pakistan of 1947 had two different territories separated by India—one to the western side of India and other to the east, known as West Pakistan and East Pakistan respectively. East Pakistan was dominated by Muslims from Bengal. The political disturbances in Pakistan and a distance of more than one thousand miles made it difficult for the residents of East Pakistan to assimilate their identity with West Pakistan. There were occasional rallies for separation that, through a nine-month long 'bloody civil war' of liberation, culminated in the creation of an independent nation-state called Bangladesh in 1971,[7] assisted by India's military intervention. The creation of Bangladesh, earlier known as East Pakistan, resulted in huge migration of refugees into Indian territory. Majorly it consisted of Hindu population as Bangladesh was dominated by Muslims. The leader of this separation was Sheikh Mujibur Rahman, who is also known as the founder of Bangladesh. As India had helped Bangladesh through use of its armed forces during the civil war, India initially built healthy cooperative ties with Bangladesh and assisted in many development-related projects.

Disagreements between India and Bangladesh surrounding the issue of illegal migrants have severely disrupted the relationship. A rising Muslim population in the border areas along the North-Eastern region of India, primarily in the state of Assam, has concerned Assam's state government. It has affected political dynamics of the Indian state of Assam. The Indian government had committed through its election manifesto in 2014 that they would tackle the problem of illegal migrants on priority basis and if the need be, would direct them to go back to Bangladesh. As a fallout, in July 2018, the government of the state of Assam published the final draft of National Register of Citizens of Assam, in which an estimated four million people living in a border area of India have been left off a controversial citizenship list designed to stem the illegal flood of immigrants from neighboring Bangladesh, the majority of them Muslim, as reported by *The Washington Post*.[8]

India, Pakistan, and Bangladesh are three independent countries and are all listed in the top 10 most populous countries of the world—India is second, Pakistan sixth, and Bangladesh eighth. The residents of West Bengal (Indian state) draw proximity in language and culture with the residents of Bangladesh. Similarly, such closeness of culture and language is observed among the residents of Punjab, Jammu and Kashmir (Indian states), and the residents of neighboring Pakistan. According to the Indian Constitution, as adopted in 1950, it is the largest multiparty participatory democracy in the world. The preamble of the Constitution provides fundamental assurances by

---

[7] For details see Tan and Kudaisya (2000), Bose and Jalal (2004) mention that '*A third war in 1971, preceded by the slaughter of Muslims by Muslims, marked the breakaway of Bangladesh*' (p. 157).

[8] Accessed from The Washington Post website on Sept 15, 2018 https://www.washingtonpost.com/world/asia_pacific/indias-muslim-migrants-fear-deportation-after-4-million-are-left-off-citizens-list/2018/07/30/0d5c28fc-bbd7-4934-821c-17e9520c0d60_story.html?noredirect=on&utm_term=.c777a9db0676.

the government towards its commitment to fairness to its citizens. All the policies in the country are drafted and implemented within the broader premise of the Constitution, assuring justice and well-being to all citizens across its states. It is visible through the progress trajectory of India that it has been able to maintain the spirit of a vibrant democracy. India has led the process of socio-economic development in the region and has been able to establish institutional democracy through its pluralistic approach. Unlike Pakistan and Bangladesh which have been under military rule a few times, India being the largest democracy of the region, has never been under military rule, which is a positive sign in assuring fair governance to its citizens. Pakistan has experienced recurrent periods of political turmoil since its independence; it took 23 years after independence to hold the first general election. Bangladesh, the youngest nation of the region, has also suffered from political problems ever since its inception. There have been further setbacks for both of these countries, as they lacked strong leadership at the time of their foundation.

India's first prime minister, Jawaharlal Nehru, who was sworn in on August 15, 1947, spearheaded the process of development for 17 years (August 15, 1947 to May 27, 1964). This process of development included the creation of facilitating infrastructure, building institutions for assuring good education, health and governance, leading towards assurance of HWB. He had a keen interest in the philosophy of socialism and his political ideas were heavily influenced by J. M. Keynes and Bertrand Russell, as he attended their lectures while in Cambridge. Further, his philosophies leaned towards the teachings of socialists like Marx and Lenin. The initiatives undertaken by the communists in the Union of Soviet Socialist Republics (USSR) to fight poverty, disease, and illiteracy impressed Nehru and helped him formulate his own public policies for the planned development of India following a mixed economic structure which had two different sides to it—participation of state in the running of enterprises and looking after the welfare of citizens. Through such infrastructure Nehru wished to establish a socialistic pattern of society. Some of the state-owned enterprises[9] were created during his leadership primarily in the areas of transportation, electricity, healthcare, education, and science and technology. He called upon the nation to build new temples of resurgent India which included building dams for irrigation, steel plants, aluminum plants, zinc plants, and more. These public work projects crowned him as the father of modern India. India thus had a steady start for its socio-economic development and this path was followed by subsequent governments. It was in the earlier part of 1990s that India became part of the World Trade Organization (WTO) and liberalized its markets. The initiatives for liberalization, globalization, and privatization of the Indian economy and market, contributed to the improvements in socio-economic indicators.

Located in the Indian Ocean (between Bay of Bengal and Arabian Sea), Sri Lanka is an island country which was first known as Ceylon. It has an ethnic, cultural, and linguistic proximity with the residents of the state of Tamil Nadu (Indian State). It

---

[9]In India state-owned enterprises are also known as public sector undertakings. These undertakings are government owned companies and function under the control of provincial government or central government as the case may be.

was ruled by the Portuguese, the Dutch and the British for around 450 years, roughly 150 years each. Ceylon gained independence from the British in 1948 and the island was renamed as Sri Lanka in 1972. The Sri Lankan population is mainly Buddhist (70%), adhering to the Theravada school, which is considered to be the most ancient form of Buddhism. The rest of the population practices either Hinduism, Islam, or Christianity. Sri Lankans primarily speak Sinhalese and Tamil, though English is also an official language. The rivalry between the Tamil and the Sinhalese has led to internal conflict and violence (Spencer, 1990). Initially, Sri Lankan public policy was predominantly socialist. It was during the later part of 1970s when Sri Lanka adopted a free market model. Sri Lanka's free market system and ensuing social progress is a model that other South Asian nations admire and hope to emulate.

The history of each of the other South Asian countries—Afghanistan, Bhutan, Nepal, and the Maldives—is different. Afghan independence was secured in 1921 after three wars with the British. Unrest in Afghanistan continued until a coup in 1973 that ended the reign of King Muhammad Zahir Shah. It shares its boundaries with Pakistan, Iran, Turkmenistan, Uzbekistan, and Tajikistan. A close relationship with the USSR followed the Saur Revolution in 1978, and the Soviet invasion of Afghanistan in 1979 resulted in an Afghani civil war. In 1989, the withdrawal of the Soviets left Afghanistan's urban cities under government control, whereas the countryside went under the control of Muslim fundamentalists. It is one of the least developed countries of South Asia, as well as in the rest of the world. Primarily, it has an agrarian economy focusing on pomology, as the farmers grow high quality of pomegranates, apricots, melons, grapes, and dry fruits. It is likely the world's largest producer of opium. Afghanistan has been infamously known for Talibani extremism[10] which has stunted development and resulted in significant loss of life—apart from the resulting destruction to physical infrastructure. Human development in Afghanistan is negatively impacted by these disturbances.

The Kingdom of Bhutan (as it is known today), is located in the Himalayan region, sandwiched between the two most populous countries in the world—China and India. It is the youngest democracy in the world, as its first general election took place in 2008. Recently, third general elections were held and the new government was formed in November 2018. Bhutan is a predominantly Buddhist nation with a total population of less than one million people. It has never been colonized by any other nation. In 1907, the governor of Trongsa, Sir Ugyen Wangchuk, was elected as the first king of Bhutan. "On 8th January 1910, the treaty of Punakha was signed and Bhutan agreed to be guided by the advice of the British Government in regard to its external relations" (Phuntsho, 2013, p. 527). It was also agreed that the British should not interfere in the internal affairs of Bhutan, albeit some violations of this agreement took place between 1910 and 1947. When British left India after India's independence in 1947, its ties with Bhutan in respect of guiding Bhutan's external relations were replaced by India. India provided both financial and operational support to help Bhutan maintain her sovereignty, peace, and order along its northern border with

---

[10] See   https://www.hrw.org/sites/default/files/world_report_download/201801world_report_web.pdf.

China. In order to provide smooth governance to its citizens, some of the important institutions were established, such as National Assembly (1953), Royal Bhutan Army (1958), and High Court (1967). Bhutan became a member of the United Nations (UN) in 1971 and it was in 1972 when the King of Bhutan spoke about the importance of gross national happiness (GNH) at a United Nations session in Geneva.

The Gorkha ruler Prithvi Narayan Shah conquered the Kathmandu valley and laid the foundation of a unified kingdom named Nepal in 1768. His expansion spree was halted by a Chinese presence in Tibet in 1792, who ruled until 1816 when the Anglo-Nepalese war was fought, and Nepal became a quasi-British protectorate. Though Nepal was never colonized by British, it had an alliance with British Empire. It functioned as a buffer state between China and India. From 1846 to 1950, members of the Rana dynasty served as hereditary chief ministers and ruled, reducing the king (Shah dynasty) to a figurehead. Anti-Rana forces based in India formed an alliance with the king, Gyanendra Bir Bikram Shah, and in 1951 the sovereignty of the crown was restored when the Nepali Congress Party (NCP) formed the government. Under Nepal's monarchical structure, the first multiparty election took place in 1959, resulting in the victory of the NCP. It was not even a year when king Mahendra seized power and control by suspending the parliament and drafting a new constitution which enforced a non-party system of councils (*panchayats*) that gave sole power to the king. In 1962, Nepal was declared a Hindu state through its constitution under the rule of king. The next 28 years saw many violent protests demanding democracy which disturbed the socio-political fabric of the country. It was during this period (1960–1988) that a 20-year health plan was implemented, and a new educational plan was introduced.

The last decade of the 20th century brought hope to the citizens of Nepal. By the end of the 1990s, a new democratic constitution was announced, and in 1991, the NCP won in the first democratic election and Girija Prasad Koirala became the prime minister. Those hopes were shattered after the Maoist movement began in 1996 in the name of a People's War.[11] The Himalayan nation experienced revolving assertions of power and control by two powerful factions, between the democratically elected government and king Mahendra. In 2008, the monarchy was finally abolished by the first Constituent Assembly. The legislative government in Nepal is called Federal Parliament and consists of two houses—the House of Representatives and the National Assembly. It has an independent Supreme Court, headed by the Chief Justice of Nepal, seven high courts, and a large number of trial courts spread across the country. Political instability and uncertainty have taken its toll on development plans. In February 2018, Prime Minister Khadga Prasad Oli (President of the NCP) was elected and new development plans for Nepal are underway. India has historically been a strong development partner for Nepal and continues to be so today.

The Maldives is the smallest country in the South Asian region, both in its size (300 km^2) and population (436,000). Located in the Indian Ocean, it has a meagre share of around 0.0002% of world's landmass and 0.01% of the total land encompassed in the South Asian region, with a population of around half a million citizens.

---

[11] For details, see Verma and Navlakha (2007).

Culturally, it is the most homogeneous state in South Asia as it has a common religion (Islam) and a common language (Divehi), both of which give the country a strong national identity. Until 1887, it was ruled by a sultan. From 1887 to 1965, the Maldives islands remained under British rule as self-governed protectorate. In 1965, the Maldives achieved full political independence. In 1968, the ad-Din sultanate was abolished in favor of a republican system of government, and Ibrahim Nasir was elected as its first president. The office of the president has extensive executive powers as he appoints the cabinet, which is approved by the People's Majlis (the unicameral legislative body or parliament). There is no provision for the separation of power and the judges are independent, subject to the constitution and law only. Wherever the constitution is silent, the judge must then consider Islamic Shariah. Maumoon Abdul Gayoom ruled the country for 30 long years, from 1978 to 2008. His office implemented multiple reforms targeted towards improving the quality of life of people, developing infrastructure, and improving trade and industry. However, the Maldives suffered setbacks due to political interventions as well as natural disasters like tsunamis. Tourism has been one of the key contributors to the Maldives' economic development.

South Asia has emerged as a promising and vibrant region for its economic development in the last decades of the 20th century and the early 21st. In 2008, *The Economist* published a story on India stating that it is on the path to becoming a tiger economy.[12] As mentioned earlier, South Asia is characterized as a group of countries with wide religious, cultural, and linguistic diversity. On one hand it has been a strength of the region, on the other, it has also posed a greater challenge in sustaining its diversity. There have been ethnic disputes and conflicts that have brought tensions of different kind, size, and complexity resulting in demand of separation. When the greater part (present-day India, Pakistan, and Bangladesh) of South Asia became independent after the colonial period ended, aspirations soared as the independence movement had built a strong sense of identity, togetherness, and cooperation. The priorities of respective governments in India, Pakistan, and Bangladesh were set to develop physical infrastructure, industry, and institutions to address issues concerning physical well-being. Bhutan and the Maldives were slower than other countries of the region. Nepal and Afghanistan were toiling hard to maintain peace. Sri Lanka was developing better as compared to other countries of the region. Overall for the South Asia region the developmental growth remained slow till around 1980. South Asia's dependence on neighboring countries and external support for development continued mounting over successive years. As compared to other parts of the world, this region started feeling the pressure of slow social and human progress which necessitated the need for broad policy shift. The last decade of the 20th century delivered promising growth in economic well-being. Generally, respective governments in the region were able to build confidence among the masses, yet economic

---

[12]See March 8, 2008 issue of *The Economist* (India Becoming a Tiger) weekly titled a story and provided arguments as to how India shall become a tiger economy. Tigers are part of Asian symbolism indicating fast economic growth leading to improving standard of living. South Korea, Taiwan, Hong Kong, and Singapore have been termed as Four Asian Tigers.

growth could not improve social indicators in the similar way. This has posed a significant challenge for the whole region. Other regions have grown much faster as compared to South Asia. Hence the necessity for exploring the reason behind this with the help of growth stories, indicators, and data to suggest future policy priorities.

There have been several cases of ethnic and communal violence within and between South Asian countries, resulting in stunted growth and development. These clashes persist despite the gradual separation from India of the recently autonomous nations of Bangladesh (formerly East Pakistan) and Pakistan, which were previously territories within historic India. The struggles between Pakistan and India in the politically divided territory of Kashmir illustrate the magnitude of the unresolved tensions that exist within South Asia on a larger scale (Uppsala Conflict Data Program, 2015), especially those recurrent confrontations between the region's two nuclear states—India and Pakistan (Ganguly & Kapur, 2012, p. 27).

Afghanistan has faced many challenges in dealing with the Kabul Marxists and the Soviet occupation. Bhutan and Nepal have never been conquered or colonized by a foreign force. Since they are sandwiched between two of the most populous nations in the world, China and India, they struggle to maintain peace and security in an otherwise conflict-ridden region. Afghanistan, Pakistan, Nepal, and Sri Lanka have a myriad of internal problems that continually hinder their progress. India's friendly relations with Nepal and Bhutan have promoted free movement across borders and have helped these countries to obtain both goods and services as well as the chance to explore opportunities that can contribute to improving their indicators of social well-being. The problems and challenges within this geographically, ethnically, culturally, and linguistically diverse region have affected relationships among these countries. The clash of civilizations within South Asia threatens the unity of the entire region and, as a result, has affected HWB. Poverty trends have improved and over the years more and more people are joining the work force. This region has the opportunity to capitalize on its available resources and follow inclusiveness in its policy to improve HWB.

1.5 South Asian Association for Regional Cooperation: A Unifying Agency

In order to establish its identity and to exploit its resources to its advantage, the nations comprising the South Asian region created the South Asian Association for Regional Cooperation (SAARC). The seed for the creation of SAARC was sown in 1981 when the foreign secretaries of seven of the South Asian countries (except Afghanistan, which became part of the group later) met in Colombo (Sri Lankan capital) in April 1981. In 1985, seven independent South Asian countries—Bangladesh, Bhutan, India, the Maldives, Nepal, Pakistan, and Sri Lanka—formed the SAARC to strengthen mutual cooperation and resource sharing in agriculture, rural development, telecommunication, meteorology, health, and population activities. The primary objective of SAARC, as defined in its charter, was to promote the welfare of the people of the region and to help improve their quality of life in addition to boosting economic growth and socio-cultural cooperation and development. SAARC also promoted mutual collaboration and assistance in economic, social, cultural, technical, and scientific arenas. As the organization grew, it kept adding more territories and objectives to its mission. In 2007, Afghanistan also joined SAARC, which made it a collation of eight countries.

In 2004, all of the member countries of SAARC signed a social charter that defined its goals of eradicating poverty, stabilizing population growth, empowering women, mobilizing youth, developing human resources, protecting children, and promoting health and nutrition. The purpose was to assure the well-being of the people of South Asia by coordinating efforts and resources to reach these goals. The policies and performance of the countries of South Asia in the domains of health, education, governance, income, life satisfaction, etc. are discussed in different chapters of this monograph.

Over the last three and half decades, SAARC has become a vibrant organization, engaging in varied initiatives to ensure increased quality of life and improved well-being for its member countries.[13] SAARC is a member of other major regional and international organizations. It operates using an important instrument called the *Integrated Plan of Action* and has various coordination committees supervising all of the nations of the region. To boost trade and commerce, and to improve the gross domestic product (GDP) in the region, the member countries have all signed the SAARC Preferential Trading Arrangement, which allows the inter-nations movement of more than 5000 commodities. The SAARC Food Security Reserve was initiated to meet the emergent nutritional needs of the member countries. The South Asian Development Fund was created to finance industrial development, poverty alleviation programs, environmental protection programs, and to protect against the problem of imbalance between import and export. SAARC has also made committed efforts to deal with gender-related issues, child welfare and development, and health and education related issues. It has signed various agreements with other concerned agencies to improve the well-being of the citizens residing in the region. Examining the history of this region and at unifying institutions such as SAARC, it could be stated that SAARC has significantly contributed to the overall development of the region as well as maintaining its identity as an effective institution to represent all countries of the South Asia region. Its contribution to improving living conditions and HWB has been immense, which shall be discussed in the following chapters.

1.6   Chapter Briefs

This book on human well-being and policy in South Asia is spread over five chapters. The nature of data used throughout the book is secondary, as it is often published

---

[13]SAARC is involved in the development activities in the areas of Human Resource Development and Tourism; Agriculture and Rural Development; Environment, Natural Disasters and Biotechnology; Economics, Trade and Finance; Social Affairs; Information and Poverty Alleviation; Energy, Transport, Science and Technology; and Education, Security and Culture. Accessed from http://saarc-sec.org/areas_of_cooperation.

in different reports such as the Human Development Report, World Development Report, World Bank Report, etc. Available published data after 1990 is used for comparisons and conclusions. Wherever comparable data for given year is not available, most approximate years' data is taken for the purpose. Major policy initiatives as reported by respective governments, funding agencies, civil society, etc. are also referred and used.

This chapter acts as the introduction to the volume which provides basic historic, geographic, socio-economic, and political profiles of all eight countries of the South Asian region, as well as a brief sketch detailing the inception, activities, and role of SAARC as an effective unifying institution for the region. The case for human well-being is defended briefly and the role of public policy in improving human well-being is outlined.

Chapter 2 introduces and provides a comparative analysis of the indicators (variables) used in the volume, namely Human Development Index, education, health, poverty, governance, life satisfaction, etc. This chapter includes a few important success stories of individuals and institutions that have worked for or influenced human well-being.

Chapter 3 examines major policy interventions which have had a positive effect on improving indicators of human well-being. It discusses the monetary allocation for health and education out of GDP and policies related to poverty alleviation, economic growth, employment, health, education, and governance. Policy comparisons and challenges are described in this chapter.

Chapter 4 contains a detailed discussion of human well-being policy interventions concerning different indicators as explained in the earlier chapters and as adopted in South Asian countries individually as well as in the region jointly. Key outcomes are analyzed wherever possible.

Chapter 5 is the concluding chapter and highlights the major takeaways of the work and guidelines for future policy direction.

References

Agrawala, S., Ota, T., Ahmed, A. U., Smith, J., & Aalst, M. V. (2003). *Development and climate change in Bangladesh: Focus on coastal flooding and the Sundarbans*. Paris: OECD. Retrieved from http://www.oecd.org/env/cc/21055658.pdf.

Bose, S., & Jalal, A. (2004). *Modern South Asia—History, culture, political economy* (2nd ed.). London: Routledge.

Chakrabarti, R., & Sanyal, K. (2017). *Public policy in India. Oxford India short introductions*. New Delhi: Oxford University Press.

Dewan, A. M., Nishigaki, M., & Komatsu, M. (2003). Floods in Bangladesh: A comparative hydrological investigation on two catastrophic events. *Journal of the Faculty of Environmental Science and Technology, 8*(1), 53–62. Retrieved from https://core.ac.uk/download/pdf/12549250.pdf.

Estes, R. J., & Sirgy, M. J. (2017). The history of well-being in global perspective. In R. J. Estes & M. J. Sirgy (Eds.), *The pursuit of human well-being—The untold global history* (pp. 691–741). Switzerland: Springer International Publishing.

Ganguly, S., & Kapur, P. (2012). *India, Pakistan, and the bomb: Debating nuclear stability in South Asia*. New York: Columbia University Press.

Gasper, D. (2004). *Human well-being: Concepts and conceptualizations*. Discussion Paper 2004/06. World Institute for Development Economics Research. Retrieved from https://www.wider.unu.edu/sites/default/files/dp2004-006.pdf.

Green, D. (2012). *From poverty to power: How active citizens and effective states can change the world* (2nd ed.). Rugby: Practical Action Publishing and Oxford.

Hofer, T., & Messerli, B. (2006). *Floods in Bangladesh: History, dynamics and rethinking the role of the Himalayas*. New York: United Nations University Press.

Huq, S. (2002). *Lessons learned from adaptation to climate change in Bangladesh*. Discussion paper. Washington DC: Environment Department, World Bank. Retrieved from https://unfccc.int/files/cooperation_and_support/capacity_building/application/pdf/bangadapt.pdf.

Kaplan, R. D. (2010). *South Asia's geography of conflict*. Washington DC: Center for a New American Security. Retrieved from https://www.cnas.org/publications/reports/south-asias-geography-of-conflict.

Kumar, P., & Narayan, S. (2007). *Sink or swim: Why disaster risk reduction is central to surviving floods in South Asia*. Briefing note. Retrieved August 18, 2015, from https://policy-practice.oxfam.org.uk/publications/sink-or-swim-why-disaster-risk-reduction-is-central-to-surviving-floods-in-sout-114596.

Mohammad-Arif, A. (2014). Introduction, imaginations and constructions of South Asia: An enchanting abstraction? *South Asia Multidisciplinary Academic Journal*. Online publication https://doi.org/10.4000/samaj.3800.

Muni, S. D. (1979). India and regionalism in South Asia: A political perspective. In B. Prasad (Ed.), *India's foreign policy: Studies in continuity and change* (pp. 105–124). New Delhi: Vikas Publishing House.

Oxfam International. (2008). *Rethinking disasters: Why death and destruction is not nature's fault but our failure*. New Delhi: Oxfam.

Petraglia, M. D., & Boivin, N. (2014). Homosapiens societies—South Asia. In V. Cummings, P. Jordan, & M. Zvelebil (Eds.), *The Oxford handbook of the archaeology and anthropology of hunter-gatherers* (pp. 328–345). Oxford: Oxford University Press.

Phuntsho, K. (2013). *The history of Bhutan*. Noida: Random House India.

Raychaudhuri, T. (1985). Historical roots of mass poverty in South Asia—A hypothesis. *Economic and Political Weekly, 20*(18), 801–806.

Roy, R. (2010). *South Asian partition fiction in English—From Khushwant Singh to Amitav Ghosh*. Amsterdam: Amsterdam University Press.

Sanyal, S. (2012). *Land of the seven rivers—A brief history of India's geography*. New Delhi: Penguin Books.

Schiermeier, Q. (2014). Floods: Holding back the tide. *Nature, 508*(7495), 164–166. https://doi.org/10.1038/508164a.

Shrotryia, V. K. (2013). Culture, gross national happiness and disasters: Strategies for preparedness and management of disasters in Bhutan. *Journal of Integrated Disaster Risk Management, 3*(1), 170–183. https://doi.org/10.5595/idrim.2013.0039.

Spencer, J. (1990). Introduction: The power of the past. In S. Jonathan (Ed.), *Sri Lanka—History and the roots of conflict* (pp. 1–18). London: Routledge.

Tan, T. Y., & Kudaisya, G. (2000). *The aftermath of partition in South Asia. Routledge studies in the modern history of Asia*. London: Routledge.

Uppsala Conflict Data Program (UCDP). (2015). *UCDP conflict encyclopedia:* www.ucdp.uu.se/database. Uppsala: Uppsala University. Retrieved August 15, 2015, from http://www.ucdp.uu.se/gpdatabase/gpcountry.php?id=74&regionSelect=6-Central_and_Southern_Asia#.

Verma, A. S., & Navlakha, G. (2007). People's war in Nepal: Genesis and development. *Economic and Political Weekly, 42*(20), 1839–1843.

World Bank. (2000). *Bangladesh climate change and sustainable development* (Report No. 21104-BD). Rural Development Unit South Asia Region. Accessed from http://documents.worldbank.org/curated/en/906951468743377163/pdf/multi0page.pdf.

Chapter 2
Human Well-Being Indicators in South Asia Region

The five ornaments of a country are health, wealth, crops, happiness and security.[a]

Abstract This chapter discusses the outcomes of public policy implementation from all of the eight countries of the South Asian region. In some cases, finding data consistency and availability has been a challenge, but overall it is consistent. Primarily, data from World Bank reports and databases across 1990–2017 are used. GDP (growth and per capita trends), health (life expectancy, infant mortality rate, survival to 65 years of age, availability of doctors and beds), education (literacy rate, mean and expected years of schooling), human development (Human Development Index), poverty (Multidimensional Poverty Index), unemployment (youth and total), and subjective well-being or happiness (life satisfaction, happy life years, World Happiness Report rankings) are tracked for the given period and comparisons are made through graphical depiction and narration in order to examine trends in each area. After reading this chapter, the reader will gain a clear understanding of the status of human well-being indicators in each country in South Asia and of the region as a whole. It would also help the reader to have a comparative view of South Asia region vis-à-vis other regions of the world. In addition, these outcomes are expected to provide appropriate guidelines for future policy direction.

Keywords Human well-being · South Asia · GDP · Health · Education · Governance · Subjective well-being · Happiness

---

[a][Thiruvalluvar] Thiruvalluvar was a great Tamil saint, poet and philosopher who wrote Thirukkural during 4th century BC, having 133 chapters of 10 couplets each, providing lessons for art of living. It has been translated in many languages. The present verse (chapter 74, verse 738) is taken from the translation done by Rajaram (2009, p. 151).

© Springer Nature Switzerland AG 2020
V. K. Shrotryia, *Human Well-Being and Policy in South Asia*, Human Well-Being Research and Policy Making, https://doi.org/10.1007/978-3-030-33270-9_2

2.1 Introduction

Quality of life, fulfillment of human needs, well-being, welfare, and happiness, are all terms often used interchangeably. All of these terms lead towards the attainment of human well-being. Before we proceed to examine the indicators of HWB, it is important that we look at the definitions of these terms for clarity. Quality of life is defined by Vaarama and Pieper (2014) as "an extent to which persons enjoy a good life by achieving a balance in their relations with themselves and with others through creating and sustaining adequate conditions and own potentials over the life course" (p. 5269). Human needs are commonly attributed to the drivers behind peoples' actions, or the motives behind human behavior (Guillen-Royo, 2014, p. 3027). Their fulfillment results in the improvement of quality of life, also known as well-being. "Well-Being is what is achieved by someone living a life that is good for him or her" (Tiberius, 2014, p. 7110). The responsibility of the state is to look after the welfare of its citizens which is defined by Wagle and Koirala (2014) as "the utility or satisfaction derived from consumption or any other economic activity such as resource allocation, trade, or distribution" (p. 7030). Satisfaction stemming from government policies and gained through using services provided by the state, enhances life satisfaction of individuals which is used as a proxy for happiness. Happiness is defined by Veenhoven (1984a) as "the degree to which a person evaluates the overall quality of his/her own life as a whole positively. In other words, how much one likes the life one lives" (p. 22). Happiness, life satisfaction, fulfillment of human needs, well-being, and subjective well-being are interrelated terms and ultimately relate to quality of life. Yet they are highly contested constructs (Phillips, 2006, p. 15).

In the present work, HWB is evaluated in terms of education well-being, health well-being, good governance, economic well-being and subjective well-being. Each of these items are tracked through different indicators such as human development, literacy rate, infant mortality rate, life expectancy, corruption index, per capita income, poverty levels, happiness levels, etc. Hence, HWB is considered to be a reflection of overall positive life condition encompassing health, education, income, happiness and good governance. It assumes people to live in harmony with each other and to lead a happy life. This chapter discusses broad outcome indicators such as human development, health status, educational conditions, trends in governance, and subjective well-being, across all eight countries falling in the South Asian region. The chapter also intends to provide a description of the aforementioned indicators as consequence of state programs and policies which are discussed in Chap. 3.

2.2 Human Development and South Asia

With numerous welfare measures in place and government concern for human progress, as reflected through public policy, there is a resulting clear improvement in human living conditions. The separate efforts of national income economists led to a commonly held belief that measurable economic progress will take care of social progress as well. In almost all parts of the world, policy frameworks were designed to attain economic progress by producing measurable outcomes which resulted in an increase of per capita income for most parts of the world. Even in some of the high-income countries corresponding improvements in social indicators were not achieved. Brazil (which was considered high income country in 1990 when first Human Development report was published) had a per capita income of USD 2020, whereas its average life expectancy was only 65 years, adult literacy rate was 78%, and infant mortality rate was 62 (per '000 live births). Similarly, in South Arabia, the per capita income was USD 6200 but average life expectancy was 64 years, adult literacy rate was 55%, and infant mortality rate was 70 (per '000 live births). On the contrary, Sri Lanka (which fell in the category of modest income country) had a per capita income of a meagre USD 400, yet it had a better average life expectancy (71 years), adult literacy rate (87%), and infant mortality rate (32 per '000 live births).[1] It was through the concerted efforts of Mahbub ul Haq[2] (former Finance and Planning Minister of Pakistan) supported by Amartya Sen, that the UN through the United Nations Development Program (UNDP), commissioned the first Human Development Report (HDR) with Mahbub ul Haq as the project director.

Box 2.1

Brief Profile of Mahbub Ul Haq

Mahbub Ul Haq is credited with the development of a statistical measurement that quantifies the indicators of economic development along with human development. He articulated a new philosophy of human development and devised the Human Development Index (HDI)[3] in 1990 which is one of the most widely used yardsticks to measure human development across a nation. HDI has been used by the United Nations Development Program for its annual Human Development Reports since then. A pioneer in economics, Haq transformed the development philosophy by shifting the focus from development as measured by national income growth to human well-being monitored through HDI. He invented the concept of people-centered development and involved scholars, policymakers, and activists to think on the same lines. His book *Reflections of human development* published in 1996[4] opened new avenues for human development paradigms. He was regarded as the

---

[1] The first Human Development Report (1990) had a mention of this data at p. 9 which provided a broader rationale for focusing on human development apart from economic growth as reflected through per capita income statistics.

[2] See Box 2.1 which provides a brief profile of Mahbub ul Haq.

[3] See https://www.britannica.com/biography/Mahbub-ul-Haq.

[4] See Haq (1996).

"most articulate and persuasive spokesman for the developing world" and named among the "top visionaries of international development"[5] by *The Economist*. During his tenure at the World Bank, his ideas and passion for human development influenced the bank's development and lending policies, poverty eradication programs, and other critical developmental issues. UNDP established the Mahbub Ul Haq Award[6] for outstanding contribution to human development in his honor. He was the Chief Economist of the Pakistan Planning Commission (1957–70), Director of the World Bank's Policy Planning Department (1970–82), Planning and Finance Minister in Pakistan's Federal Cabinet (1982–88) and Special Adviser to the UNDP Administrator (1990–96).[7] He also founded the Human Development Center in Pakistan—a policy research institute organizing professional research and policy studies in the area of human development, with focus on the South Asian region.[8] He always emphasized the importance of peace between India and Pakistan, recommended investments for education and health for all irrespective of gender, income, location, and other factors etc., in order to empower South Asian civil societies with resources and training. He relentlessly advocated for better developmental cooperation in and a system of global institutions for an integrated South Asian society. He fearlessly talked about cutting military spending to free resources for social development and endorsed a more transparent and ethical system of governance. He is known for his intellectual courage as he always fought for the marginalized and oppressed section of society against unethical and corrupt systems. His untimely death in 1998 came as a major loss to the world. Amartya Sen regarded him as an outstanding economist, a visionary thinker, global intellect and the leading architect in the contemporary world of the assessment of the process of human development.[9]

It is generally believed that human development is a process of enlarging people's choices. Though these choices are potentially unlimited, they are primarily identified as; to lead a long and healthy life (health), to acquire knowledge (education), and to have access to resources needed for a decent standard of living (income).[10] The Human Development Reports (HDRs) are published out every year to track and report human progress largely through these identified indicators. Monetary power (income) is regarded as an important component for improving quality-of-life, vis-à-vis well-being because large incomes create more opportunities for choice. However, development which only results in the increase of income, i.e., without the

---

[5] See https://www.economist.com/obituary/1998/07/23/mahbub-ul-haq.

[6] For award details see http://hdr.undp.org/en/hd-awards.

[7] See https://tribune.com.pk/story/737535/rembering-mahbubul-haq-his-work/.

[8] See https://tribune.com.pk/story/1051667/honouring-mahbubul-haq/.

[9] See https://blog.oup.com/2017/09/mahbub-ul-haq-philosophy-economics/.

[10] See UNDP (1990, p. 10).

assurance of good health and education, does not carry much weight. Good health conditions and educational empowerment are essential to make such income sustainable. Improvements in health and education indicators mark the ability of people to achieve happiness autonomously and economically sustain themselves. In one-sided efforts to boost economic growth, social progress often gets side-lined and compromised. Generally, policies are so much influenced by the achievement of short-term growth targets that social concerns unwillingly become secondary. In order to maintain a balance between economic and social progress, a policy shift was desperately needed. However, that was not possible in the absence of comparable data and convincing arguments. The initiative which assessed human progress apart from income or GDP was driven by this motivation. Ultimately what all development policies should assure is good living and improvements in HWB.

The period between 1990 and 2017 has witnessed some of the most disruptive advances in the field of technology. The use of technology has contributed towards improving physical life conditions. In addition to technology, globalization has also been a strong force driving development across the world. Globalization has created ample opportunities and influenced income positively. The globalization index generated expected favorable influence on overall HDI (Tsai, 2006) which is in agreement with the theoretical proposition projected by Sirgy, Lee, Miller, and Littlefield (2004) articulating the effect of globalization on improving the quality of human life. Individual as well as state expenditure on health and education has gained prominence resulting in improvements in health, nutrition, and literacy. Overtime, the ambit of HDI has increased to include the measurement of inequality, gender, and poverty apart from its traditional measures of health, education, and income. The purpose of reporting human progress through these important indicators is to have the ability to examine the policies at different levels in order to prioritize human development over economic development as human development is holistic in nature and also takes care of economic development.

Achieving targets for improvements in health, education, and other related parameters is only one part of the concern; the other part, which is more important, is its sustainability through consistency in policies. Reports published thus far have had some focus areas of reporting progress through sustainability, like in 1990 when the publication of HDRs started, its first report was titled "Concept and Measurement of Human Development"; and in 2016 it released a report titled "Human Development for Everyone." The emphasis on these areas (Box 2.2) provides a picture of concern on different dimensions of human progress (and vulnerabilities) which all contribute to improving quality of life and/or HWB. The reports provide an indicator (HDI) for countries to see their progress in human development, and accordingly the policies are designed to choose their priority areas of focus. The reports have been able to help pre-empt development threat areas and provide avenues to tackle these issues effectively. For example—in HDR (2014), one of the key issues raised was providing meaningful employment opportunities to all adult job-seekers—which should be embraced as a universal goal, just as education or health care is (UNDP, 2014, p. 12)—as secured employment undoubtedly provides security, satisfaction, and boosts morale and self-esteem for citizens. It creates a positive public opinion concerning the state and contributes towards building a sense of belonging and ownership for citizens. This has been one of the key areas of concern for South Asia region as well.

Box 2.2

Focus of Human Development Reports 1990–2016

1990	Concept and Measurement of Human Development
1991	Financing Human Development
1992	Global Dimensions of Human Development
1993	People's Participation
1994	New Dimensions of Human Security
1995	Gender and Human Development
1996	Economic Growth and Human Development
1997	Human Development to Eradicate Poverty
1998	Consumption for Human Development
1999	Globalization with a Human Face
2000	Human Rights and Human Development
2001	Making New Technologies Work for Human Development
2002	Deepening Democracy in a Fragmented World
2003	Millennium Development Goals: A Compact among Nations to End Human Poverty
2004	Cultural Liberty in Today's Diverse World
2005	International Cooperation at a Crossroads: Aid, Trade and Security in an Unequal World
2006	Beyond Scarcity: Power, Poverty and the Global Water Crisis
2007/2008	Fighting Climate Change: Human Solidarity in a Divided World
2009	Overcoming Barriers: Human Mobility and Development
2010	The Real Wealth of Nations: Pathways to Human Development
2011	Sustainability and Equity: A Better Future for All
2013	The Rise of the South: Human Progress in a Diverse World
2014	Sustaining Human Progress: Reducing Vulnerability and Building Resilience
2015	Work for Human Development
2016	Human Development for Everyone

The South Asian region, despite being one of the least economically developed regions in the world, has made some progress between 1991 and 2017 in human development. No country from this region is located among the top one-third of nations in terms of human development index. Sri Lanka is the only country which is bracketed in the "High Human Development" group as reflected in the HDRs. Whereas the Maldives, India, Bhutan, and Bangladesh are categorized as countries with "Medium Human Development"; and Nepal, Pakistan, and Afghanistan are placed in the "Low Human Development" category. A nation's concern for improving health and education becomes visible through these rankings, as nations are perpetually trying to improve their scores. Looking at their scores (Fig. 2.1; Table 2.1), it becomes clear that there is a significant improvement over the years. Between 1991 and 2011, among all the eight South Asian nations, Bangladesh grew fastest, followed by Nepal, India, and then Pakistan. But as Sri Lanka was already placed in the High Human Development countries category, its developmental pace was found to be comparatively slow.

There are gender differences in HDI across globe and the conditions in South Asia are even worst. Typically, females experience more problems and discrimination in education, health, work environment, etc. "Worldwide, the average HDI value for women (0.705) is 5.9% lower than that for men (0.749). Much of the gap is due to

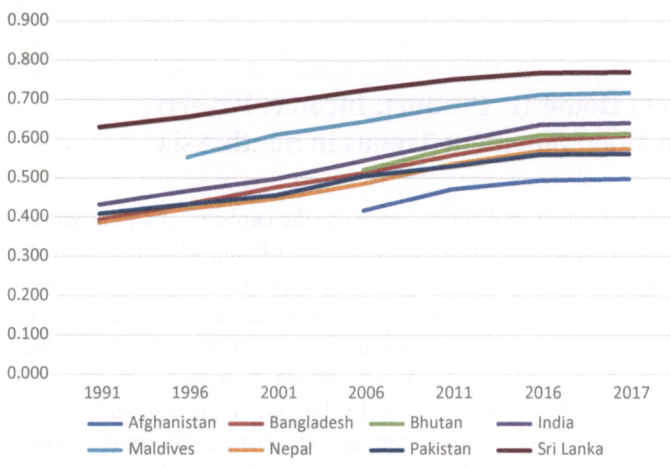

Fig. 2.1 Trends in human development index (1990–2017)

Table 2.1 Human development index values (1991–2017)

	1991	1996	2001	2006	2011	2016	2017
Afghanistan	NA	NA	NA	0.417	0.471	0.494	0.498
Bangladesh	0.394	0.433	0.477	0.513	0.557	0.597	0.608
Bhutan	NA	NA	NA	0.521	0.575	0.609	0.612
India	0.432	0.467	0.498	0.545	0.591	0.636	0.640
The Maldives	NA	0.553	0.610	0.643	0.682	0.712	0.717
Nepal	0.386	0.420	0.447	0.486	0.535	0.569	0.574
Pakistan	0.409	0.433	0.457	0.505	0.530	0.560	0.562
Sri Lanka	0.630	0.655	0.691	0.724	0.751	0.768	0.770

women's lower income and educational attainment in many countries" (UNDP, 2018, p. 5). In 2018, South Asia remained a region with the widest gender gap at 16.3% as against Latin America and the Caribbean where it is 2.3%.[11] The developmental efforts of other regions and nations around the world are much more effective than those attempted in the South Asian region to reduce this gap—as there is an improvement of 2% at the world level as compared to a meagre 0.7% improvement in South Asia. If we look at the trends in HDI overall, at 45.3%, South Asia is considered to be the fastest growing region in human development over the period of 1990–2017, followed by East Asia and the Pacific at 41.8%; and Sub-Saharan Africa at 34.9%. It could be due to its lower beginning status, enabling more scope of faster growth in the region. The impact of globalization could also be one of the reasons for this rate of growth. The policy focus of the South Asia region as discussed in Chap. 3 has been to improve human development parameters so that HWB is improved across region.

2.3   Gross Domestic Product, Income, Poverty, and Unemployment Trends in South Asia

Income is an important indicator to measure the capacity of an individual to acquire resources. It is a means to procure and enjoy well-being while also providing security for the future. While income is a prime measure of satisfaction for an individual, production is the measure of satisfaction for a nation. "Income is a means, not an end. It may be used for essential medicines or for narcotic drugs. Well-being of a society largely depends on the uses to which income is put; not on the level of income itself" (UNDP, 1990, p. 10). In the contemporary world, GDP has been considered as one of the most important indicators of the progress of a nation.[12] Economic progress has been determining the speed of development through the eyes of Kuznets (1934) and Stone[13] via production, income, and output which had its roots in Adam Smith's "invisible hand" metaphor as described in *The Theory of Moral Sentiments* and *The Wealth of Nations.*[14] Paul Samuelson and William Nordhaus viewed GDP as one of the greatest inventions of the 20th century.[15] It is believed that economic empowerment results in broadening choices and freedoms, thereby improving well-being. Though advocates of human development prioritize health

---

[11] See UNDP (2018, p. 6).

[12] A detailed note on GDP, its relevance and need for alternate measure has been provided in the concluding chapter.

[13] Richard Stone was a British economist who is also known as the father of national income accounting. He along with Kuznets, is also credited with a contribution on developing the concept of GDP based on different methods of its calculation. Both of them were noble laureates for economic sciences, Kuznets in 1971 and Stone in 1984, for their respective contributions.

[14] Adam Smith talked about *the invisible hand* first in his book *The Theory of Moral Sentiments* and then elaborated it in *The Wealth of Nations.* It is the efforts put by individuals for following self-interest but inadvertently resulting in the public good.

[15] See   https://fraser.stlouisfed.org/files/docs/publications/SCB/pages/2000-2004/35260_2000-2004.pdf.

and education over income, they too consider GDP and income as an important input for improving social infrastructure and indicators. Interestingly, it is the "invisible hand" which comes into play when it creates public good. Its role in developing regions like that of South Asia becomes more important relatively.

South Asia is a densely populated emerging economy, yet it remains one of the world's most deprived regions. As per World Bank data of 2017, this region had per capita GDP of USD 6494 (38% of world), which was only around USD 81 in 1960 (18% of world). The GDP per capita in South Asia in 1990 was USD 1194, which was 21% of the world's GDP per capita. The trend of GDP across 1960–2017 shows increasing numbers for the world as well as for the South Asian region. However, the pace of growth in South Asia was much faster during 1991–2017 as compared to the preceding period. The impact of globalization and liberalization is visible in South Asia and it has some of the fastest emerging economies of the world. Relatively, this region has grown strong economically as compared to other parts of the world, however, its problems with social infrastructure and governance have been major obstructions in the process of developing the region holistically. The region which houses around 25% of world's population, produces only 4% of world's GDP. However, it is important to remember that over the last two decades the growth has been phenomenal. As mentioned in the first chapter, South Asia region is indo-centric, India has been emerging as a dominate economy in the region for all these years (1990–2017). Though it has around 75% of the region's population, its share in GDP is much higher. Figure 2.2 depicts that in 1960 it had a 78.51% share in the GDP within the region (2.67% of world GDP), which reached 81%

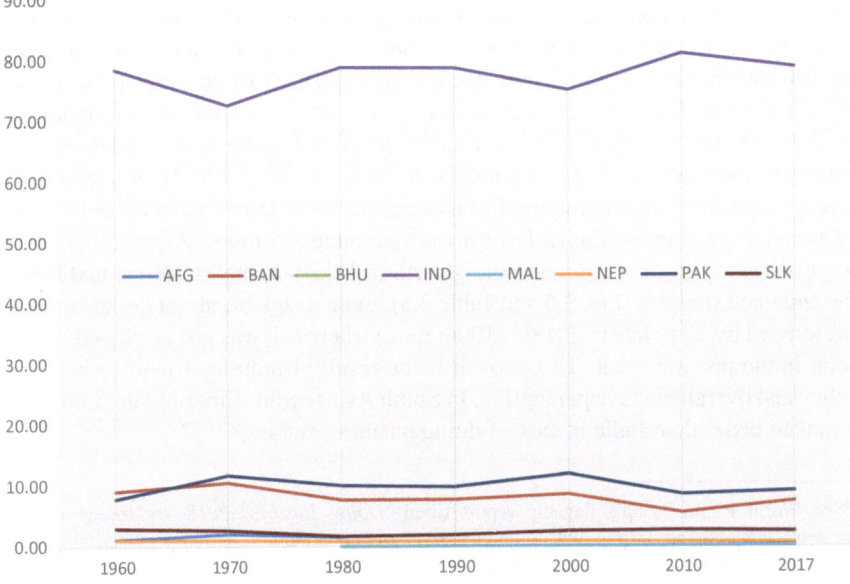

Fig. 2.2 Country-wise trends in GDP proportion (1960–2017)

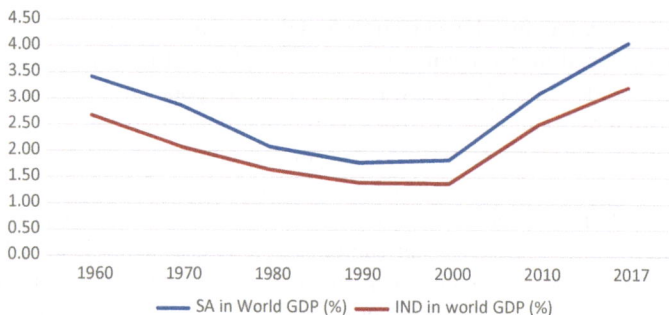

Fig. 2.3 Trends of contribution of South Asia and India in world GDP

in 2010 (2.51% of world GDP), and in 2017 it was around 79% (3.22% of world GDP). Projections are that India's share shall continue to increase further (Fig. 2.3; Table 2.2).

A comparison of GDP using 1990 prices (USD) shows that, between 1600 (the year when East India Company was founded) and 1947, the GDP for India only increased by roughly 3 times whereas for the United Kingdom it increased by more than 50 times, corresponding to a per capita increase of 1.1 times and 6.5 times, respectively. India has grown at a faster pace than other parts of the world in the last six decades. However, social indicators and outcomes have not improved in the same proportion, as per expectations. India now faces challenges to sustaining this growth and to translate it into improved citizen well-being.

The GDP per capita of South Asia has grown more than five times between 1990–2017, compared against the world growth of a little more than three times (Fig. 2.4 and Table 2.3). It shows that the growth in South Asia has been much faster in last two and a half decades as compared to the rest of the world. Though the Maldives has the highest GDP per capita across the region, making it the richest country (followed by Sri Lanka), its growth in the last two decades has not been as impressive as other countries in the region (Fig. 2.5). Bhutan and India have grown fastest by multiplying its GDP per capita by more than 6 times between 1990 and 2017, and Sri Lanka has grown by around 5.5 times. Afghanistan is the poorest country in the region and the growth in Pakistan, the Maldives, and Nepal has remained sluggish (Fig. 2.5 and Table 2.3). India's rank in ease of doing business has jumped by 30 points in 2018[16] (100th rank) whereas it was just increased by one point in the previous year. This growth is the result of industry-friendly economic policy and overall positive perception. In South Asia region, only Bhutan (75th rank) is ranked better than India in ease of doing business rankings.[17]

---

[16]See World Bank Group's flagship report titled '*Doing Business 2018—reforming to create job*' available on http://www.doingbusiness.org/content/dam/doingBusiness/media/Annual-Reports/English/DB2018-Full-Report.pdf.

[17]The ranking of other countries of the South Asia region are—Nepal 105th, Sri Lanka 111th, The Maldives 136th, Pakistan 147th, Bangladesh 177th, and Afghanistan 183th.

Table 2.2 GDP ratio in percentage

Year	In SA GDP								In world GDP	
	AFG	BGD	BTN	IND	MLD	NPL	PAK	SL	SA	IND
1960	1.16	9.19	NA	78.51	NA	1.09	7.97	3.03	3.41	2.67
1970	2.06	10.61	NA	72.70	NA	1.02	11.84	2.71	2.87	2.08
1980	1.56	7.78	0.06	78.87	0.02	0.83	10.16	1.73	2.09	1.65
1990	NA	7.86	0.07	78.77	0.05	0.90	9.95	2.00	1.78	1.40
2010	NA	8.68	0.07	75.18	0.10	0.89	12.03	2.66	1.83	1.38
2010	0.78	5.65	0.08	81.12	0.13	0.78	8.69	2.78	3.10	2.51
2017	0.63	7.59	0.08	78.91	0.14	0.74	9.26	2.65	4.08	3.22

Source Compiled from world development indicators as updated in September 2018

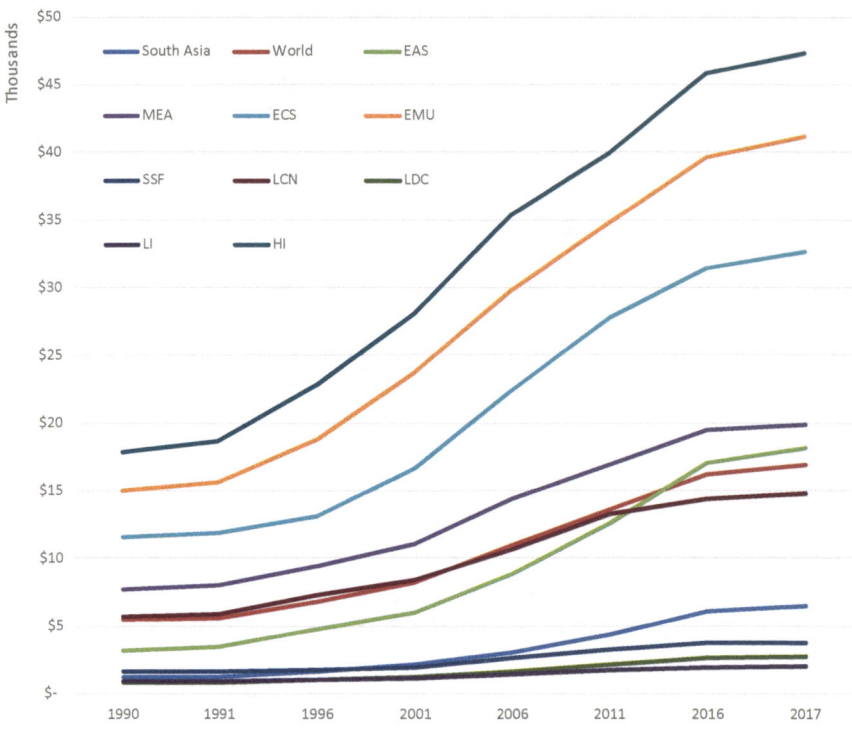

Fig. 2.4 Trends in GDP growth: world regions

Economically, East Asia and Pacific, and South Asia have grown by more than five times (1990–2017) as compared to all other regions where this growth has been much lower (Fig. 2.6). The GDP per capita in Europe and Central Asia grew by 2.82 times, OECD[18] members by 2.6 times, Middle East and North Africa by 2.58 times, and Sub-Saharan Africa grew by 2.34 times. The least developed countries recorded 3.25 times growth. During 2001–2017, the growth in India remained the fastest followed by Bhutan, which is higher than the average of the South Asian region. The per capita income in the world grew by around 2 times whereas South Asia grew by more than 3 times.

The growth of the South Asian region during the last 25 years (1993–2018) has been much faster than the growth during the preceding 32 years (1960–1992), caused by the liberalization of economics of the governments in the region. The flow of capital, through these countries and beyond, has remained positive during the last

---

[18] OECD stands for Organisation for Economic Co-operation and Development. It is a group of 36 member countries including the US, the UK, Canada, Australia, Japan, Switzerland, Italy, Germany, etc.

Table 2.3 GDP per capita growth in times

Group/region/country	1990–2017	1990–2001	2001–2011	2011–2017
Low income	**2.22**	1.21	1.54	1.19
Sub-Saharan Africa	**2.34**	1.20	1.68	1.16
Middle East and North Africa	**2.58**	1.43	1.54	1.17
OECD members	**2.61**	1.56	1.41	1.19
Latin America and Caribbean	**2.62**	1.49	1.58	1.12
High income	**2.65**	1.58	1.42	1.18
European Union	**2.74**	1.58	1.47	1.18
Pakistan	**2.80**	1.43	1.52	1.28
Europe and Central Asia	**2.82**	1.44	1.67	1.17
World	**3.11**	1.51	1.65	1.25
Least developed countries	**3.25**	1.40	1.83	1.27
Nepal	**3.46**	1.66	1.58	1.32
Bangladesh	**4.65**	1.65	1.87	1.50
South Asia	**5.44**	1.75	2.09	1.49
Sri Lanka	**5.49**	1.88	2.09	1.39
East Asia and Pacific	**5.68**	1.88	2.10	1.44
India	**6.22**	1.84	2.22	1.52
Bhutan	**6.36**	2.01	2.25	1.40

Source Compiled from World Bank database as updated on September 2018

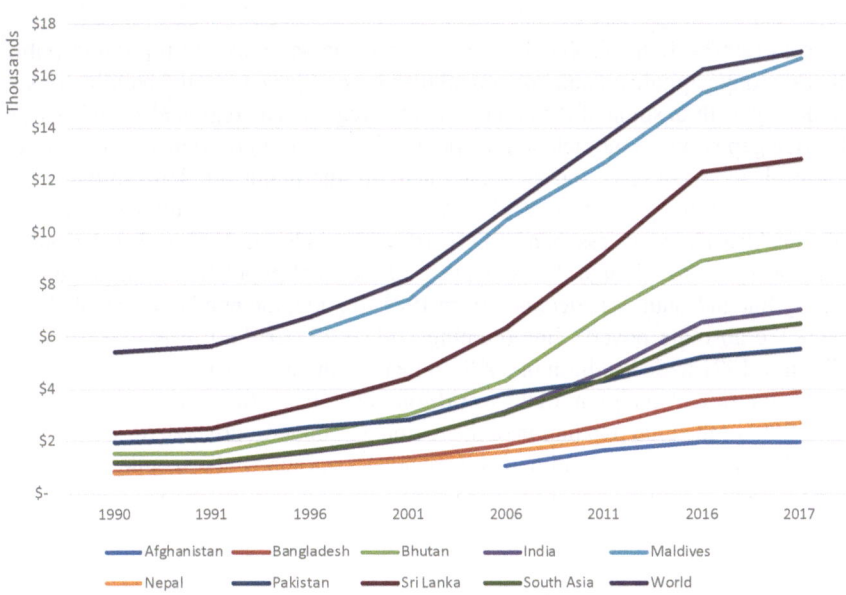

Fig. 2.5 Trends in GDP growth: South Asia Region

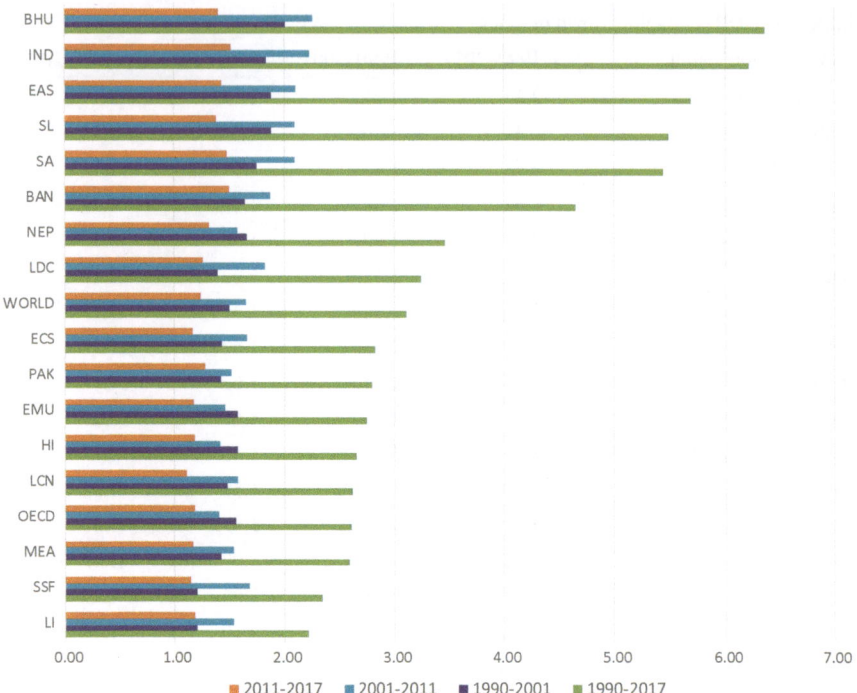

Fig. 2.6 GDP per capita growth in times (1990–2017)

15 years (2003–2018). Problems related to poor governance, corruption in public offices, crony capitalism, and communal disharmony have been the building blocks for slow growth in some of the countries in the region. The region also suffers from the wide gap between the rich and the poor reflected through extensive inequalities.

Prevalence of poverty and unemployment are the major problems in the region which has deterred growth. In 2013, 98% of the population in South Asia and Sub-Saharan Africa lived on less than USD 10 a day (World Bank, 2013, p. 58). According to the World Bank, though the percentage of the total population living below the poverty line in South Asia declined from 1981 to 2008, the number of people living below the absolute poverty line (earning USD 1.25 per day) increased from 568 million in 1981 to 571 million in 2008. In fact,South Asia has more people living in poverty than all other regions of the world combined. It is estimated that, from 2005 to 2008, 20% of the total population of the region was undernourished. In addition, one third of the adult women residing in this region were found to be anemic (Table 2.4).

Table 2.4 Multidimensional poverty index

Country	Index value	PPP USD 1.90 a day
Afghanistan	0.273	NA
Bangladesh	0.194	14.80
Bhutan	0.175	2.20
India	0.121	21.20
The Maldives	0.007	7.30
Nepal	0.154	15.00
Pakistan	0.228	6.10

Source Compiled from statistical update 2018: human development indices and indicators (UNDP 2018: Table 6)

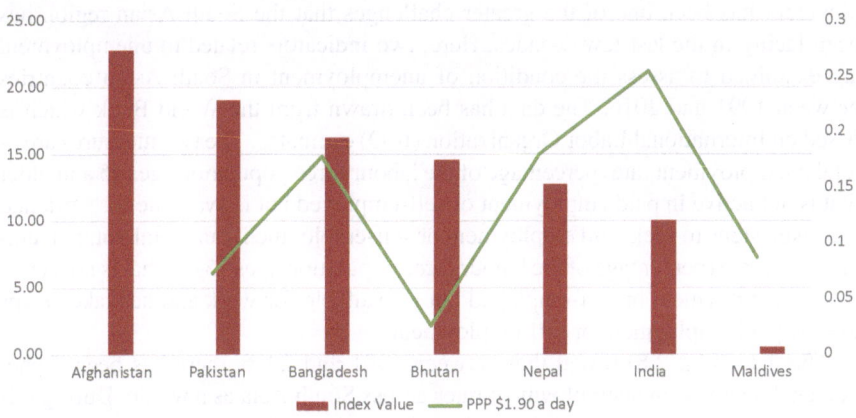

Fig. 2.7 Multidimensional poverty index in South Asian countries 2018

Multidimensional poverty[19] is found in all developing regions of the world, but it is particularly acute in Sub-Saharan Africa and South Asia. These two regions, together, account for 83% of all multi-dimensionally poor people in the world—more than 1.1 billion people. 39% of children in South Asia are multi-dimensionally poor (OPHI, 2018: x). On the world map, South Asia is the second poorest region, only slightly better than Sub-Saharan Africa in both the multidimensional poverty index (MPI) and poverty rate (OPHI, 2018, p. 45). India has the largest population of poor people as compared to other countries in South Asia. The Maldives is the richest and Afghanistan is the poorest (Fig. 2.7). Despite the many problems plaguing the region, India has performed satisfactorily in terms of economic growth. The initiatives taken up by the government in India have started reaping rich fruits. Political disturbances

---

[19]The Oxford Poverty and Human Development Initiative (OPHI) measures multidimensional poverty which is calculated on the basis of three dimensions of poverty: health (nutrition and child mortality), education (years of schooling and school attendance), and living standards (cooking fuel, sanitation, drinking water, electricity, housing, and assets).

in Pakistan, Bangladesh and the Maldives have affected their momentum of growth which has influenced the indicators of the region. The growth in other regions has been much slower as compared to the growth in this region. The investments (domestic or foreign) are on a declining trend in India and Sri Lanka but rising in other countries of the region. South Asia has least integration with other parts as its exports account only around 10% of its GDP.

Economic growth, poverty, and unemployment are closely related constructs determining public policy. Unemployment is one of the key determinants of socio-economic development which is a reflection of state policy towards improving education standards, providing skill-based education, and creating job opportunities. Creation of job opportunities has multifaceted benefits which on one side brings people to work—positively influencing production—and on the other side enhances the value of human capital, apart from reducing poverty levels. Reducing unemployment has been one of the greater challenges that the South Asian region has been facing in the last few decades. Here, two indicators related to unemployment are examined to assess the condition of unemployment in South Asian countries between 1991 and 2016. The data has been drawn from the World Bank which is based on International Labor Organization (ILO) estimates. The two measures are— total unemployment rate (percentage of the labour force population ages 15 and older that is not active in paid employment or self-employed but is available for work and has taken steps to seek paid employment or self-employment) and total youth unemployment rate (percentage of the labour force population ages 15–24 that is not active in paid employment or self-employed but is available for work and has taken steps to seek paid employment or self-employment).

The data (Fig. 2.8) reveal that between 1991 and 2016, there has been a phenomenal decrease in unemployment rates across South Asia as a whole. During this period, all of the countries of the region were trying to improve their employment conditions, to good effect. Afghanistan and Sri Lanka are worst hit nations so far as unemployment is concerned, though the reasons are distinctly different. Economic and social development in Afghanistan are the slowest in South Asia as well as in the rest of the world, which have negatively affected job opportunities. On the other side, Sri Lanka is an outlier country from this region when it comes to improvements in social indicators—health and education. It has produced more educated people than other South Asian nations but surprisingly failed to create appropriate job opportunities for them. Unemployment has been consistently on the rise in the Maldives and Bangladesh over the years, more severe in the case of youth. Education parameters in Bhutan have improved as concerted efforts were made by the government to provide education to all. It has created unemployment because corresponding increase in job opportunities has not happened. Much the same is the case with the Maldives which has not been able to increase sufficient employment avenues. Employment conditions are not very positive in India as well where though economic activities have grown and education status has also improved but it has not been able to provide employment to educated youth as expected. There have been problems of employability across India. ILO (2018, p. 2) states, "Unemployment in developing countries is expected to increase by half a million per year in both 2018 and 2019, with the

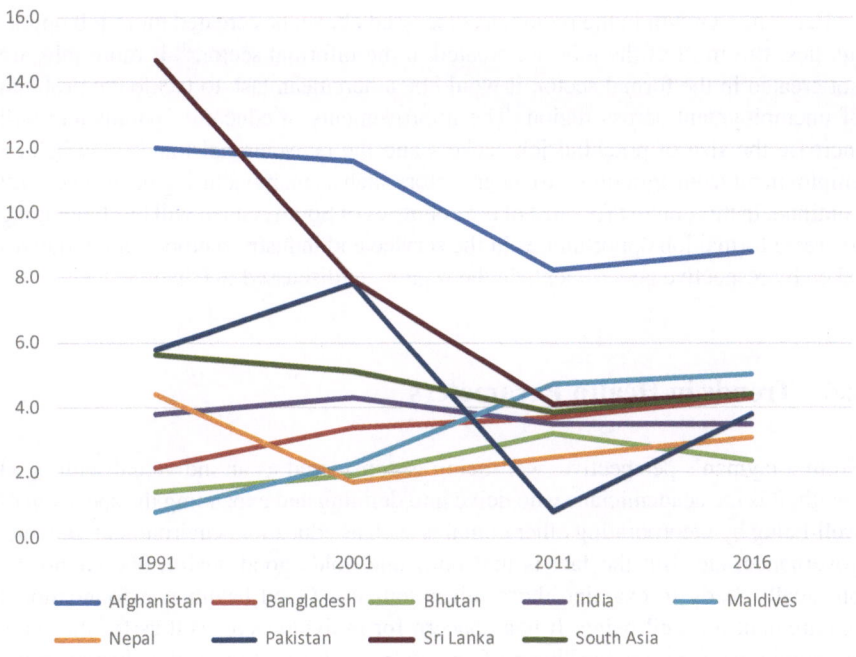

Fig. 2.8   Unemployment rate (average of total and youth)

unemployment rate remaining at around 5.3%. For many developing and emerging countries, however, persistent poor-quality employment and working poverty pose the main challenge". Focused efforts are required by all the countries of the region to boost employment opportunities (Table 2.5).

Table 2.5   Unemployment rate

Countries/region	1991		2001		2011		2016	
	Total	Youth	Total	Youth	Total	Youth	Total	Youth
Afghanistan	12.0	25.60	11.6	24.30	8.2	17.30	8.8	17.90
Bangladesh	2.2	4.50	3.4	8.60	3.7	7.30	4.3	11.10
Bhutan	1.4	3.90	1.9	5.10	3.2	9.10	2.4	10.10
India	3.8	8.50	4.3	9.90	3.5	10.30	3.5	10.50
The Maldives	0.8	1.80	2.3	5.10	4.7	10.50	5.0	13.50
Nepal	4.4	7.10	1.7	2.70	2.5	4.20	3.1	5.00
Pakistan	5.8	10.10	7.8	14.10	0.8	1.80	3.8	7.30
Sri Lanka	14.7	41.90	7.9	25.10	4.1	17.00	4.4	22.10
South Asia	**5.6**	**12.9**	**5.1**	**11.9**	**3.8**	**9.7**	**4.4**	**12.2**

Source Compiled from World Bank database as updated on September 2018

Economic growth in the region, as discussed above, has created more job opportunities. But most of the jobs are created in the informal sector.[20] If more jobs are not created in the formal sector, it would be a herculean task to tackle the problem of unemployment across region. The improvements in education parameters will increase the size of potential job seekers and the conventional trend of switching employment from agriculture to other sectors such as manufacturing or services will continue. In this context for most of the countries of South Asia, it will be challenging to create formal job opportunities in the service and industry sectors. The initiatives taken by respective governments in the region are discussed in Chap. 3.

2.4   Trends in Health Parameters

From a layman's perspective, well-being is considered as an individual with good health. It is the academicians who delve into defining and expanding the spectrum of well-being by incorporating other domains such as education, environment, income, governance, etc. But the fact is that until one holds good health, one cannot be physically ready to examine those other domains. Good health is a foundational requirement for well-being. It is a concern for individuals as well as for the state, as individuals form the backbone of any state. In this section of the chapter, some key health parameters are discussed and analyzed in order to understand the status of health in the South Asian region. Life expectancy and infant mortality rate (IMR) are two important health outcomes that are discussed with the help of data related to South Asian countries. For the purpose of analysis, the data and reports published by the UN and the World Bank are taken between 1990 and 2017.

Public health scholars agree that years of average life expectancy at birth (number of years a new-born infant could expect to live if prevailing patterns of age-specific mortality rates at the time of birth stay the same throughout the infant's life) are a major contributor to well-being and are both an indicator of the health of a country and of the quality of its health care systems. Overall health and years of average life expectancy are affected by access to health services and the quality of the services provided. Through the data available for last 70 years it is seen that in the post-World War II period, there were significant increases in life expectancy around the world, which is considered a notable achievement in the human history (Ram, 1998). This increase in the South Asian region over the last seven decades has been dramatic. The data available for 1991–2016 show that on average, the life span of a person living in this region has increased by 12 years between 1991 and 2016. Bhutan had the fastest growth adding more than 16 years to average life expectancy, followed by Nepal; the Maldives had the highest life expectancy in the region in 2016. Since Sri Lanka already had highest life expectancy in 1991, it had relatively less scope

---

[20]Informal sector is determined by the nature of job and reflects that kind of jobs that are not recognised as normal income sources and, in most cases, taxes are not paid by the workforce employed in this sector.

for increase, however it did increase its life expectancy by more than 5 years in the following 27 years. Overall if we look at the whole region, growth has been consistent. Afghanistan outperformed Pakistan, as the gap between their average life expectancy was 10 years in 1991, which drastically reduced to 3 years in 2016. Sri Lanka and the Maldives are considered outliers in terms of health parameters as their status is much better than other countries of the region (Fig. 2.9; Table 2.6).

Generally, women live longer than men in most South Asian countries, albeit life expectancy for men in the region is on the rise. As countries progress along this critical dimension of human development, the gap between the rate of survival to age 65 of both men and women is consistently increasing, quite the contrary of the world trend. Bangladesh is an exceptional country in this regard, as males have a greater life expectancy as compared to their female counterparts, though that gap is shrinking (Fig. 2.10). Over time, the conditions of gap between male-female survival to the age of 65 years have changed, and the male-female life expectancy graph has grown. On average, 89% of the women born in the Maldives in 2016 could potentially live to age 65 whereas only 85% of men born in the Maldives in 2016 are expected to reach 65—still higher than during earlier decades but the male-female gap in average years of life expectancy persists. This pattern is prevalent region wide. However, in future, as male life expectancy continues to improve, this gap will become smaller. Bangladesh has performed much better in the region in reducing this gap by improving health facilities.

IMR data reflect the quality of nutrition and hygiene during the early stages of life, which contribute to life expectancy as well. The gradual decline in the IMR

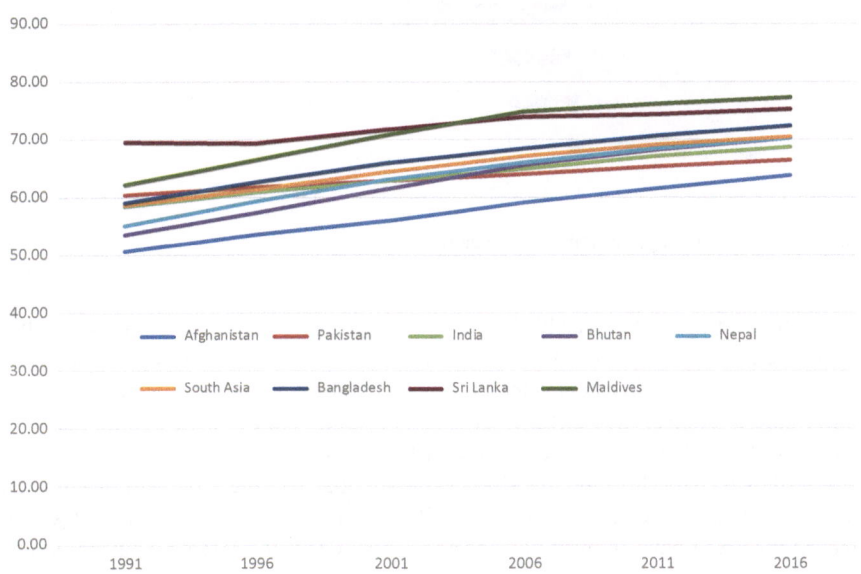

Fig. 2.9 Trends in life expectancy (in years) in South Asian countries

Table 2.6 Life expectancy in South Asia (1991–2016)

Country/region	1991	1996	2001	2006	2011	2016
Afghanistan	50.63	53.53	56.04	59.11	61.67	63.67
Bangladesh	59.03	62.61	65.90	68.40	70.63	72.49
Bhutan	53.64	57.43	61.63	65.58	68.23	70.20
India	58.41	60.88	62.98	64.97	67.01	68.56
The Maldives	62.24	66.41	70.84	74.77	76.26	77.34
Nepal	55.13	59.34	63.08	66.07	68.33	70.25
Pakistan	60.34	61.70	62.97	64.06	65.42	66.48
Sri Lanka	69.63	69.27	71.78	74.06	74.46	75.28
SA Mean	**69.63**	**69.27**	**71.78**	**74.06**	**74.46**	**75.28**

Source Compiled from World Bank database as updated on September 2018

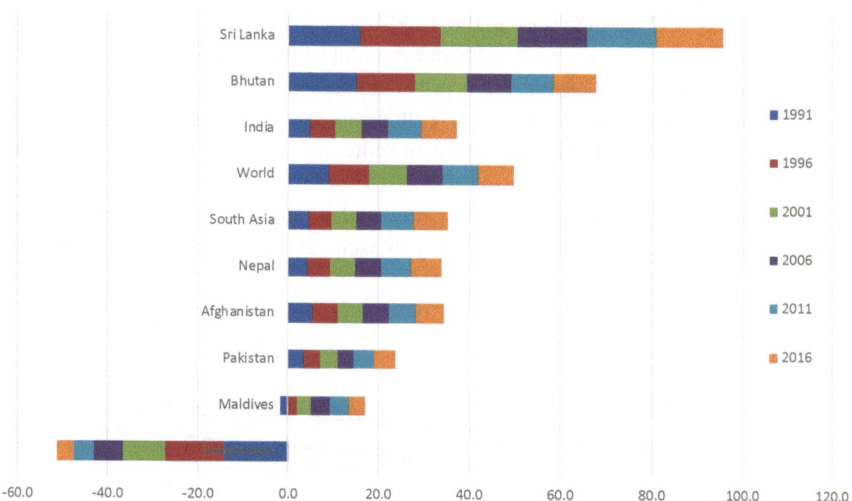

Fig. 2.10 Survival to age 65 (female-male gap)

(probability of dying between birth and exactly age 1, expressed per 1000 live births) is a reflection of policy focus towards improving the health of children. As reflected in educational and other health indicators, the Maldives, and Sri Lanka have been better able to control the mortality of infants as compared to their counterparts. In Bangladesh, the IMR has decreased the fastest between 1991 and 2017 (Fig. 2.11), followed by Nepal. The trend in India is similar to that average in the region. Pakistan had the highest IMR at 61.2 in 2017 followed by Afghanistan at 51.5. Pakistan and Afghanistan have showed poor performance. Overall, IMR for South Asia has declined, and it is expected that it will continue to further decline in the future. South Asia as a region had an IMR of 36.4 deaths per 1000 live births in 2017 compared

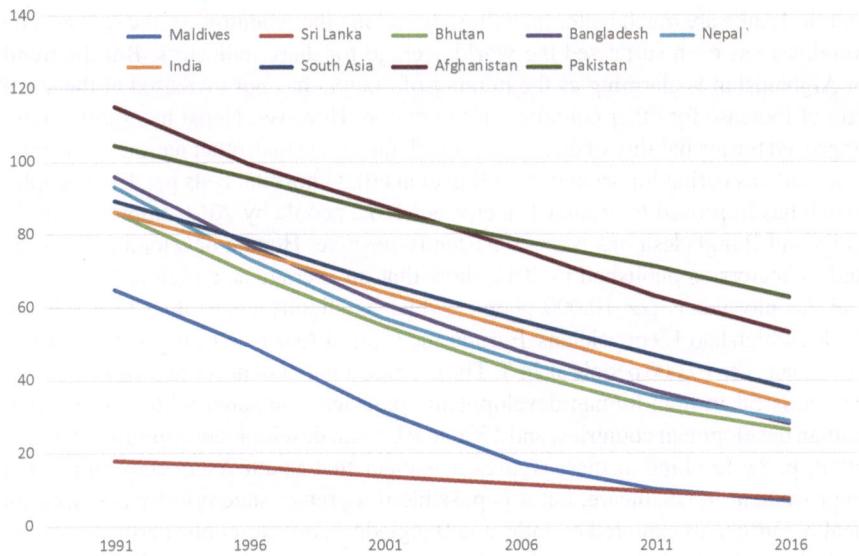

Fig. 2.11 Trends in infant mortality rate

Table 2.7 Infant mortality rate in South Asia (1991–2017)

Country/region	1991	1996	2001	2006	2011	2016	2017
Afghanistan	115.1	99.5	88.0	75.8	63.2	53.2	51.5
Bangladesh	95.9	77.3	61.0	48.0	36.9	28.3	26.9
Bhutan	86.1	69.5	55.1	42.5	32.5	26.5	25.6
India	86.3	75.8	64.4	53.7	43.2	33.6	32.0
The Maldives	65.1	49.7	31.4	17.1	10.2	7.1	6.8
Nepal	93.1	73.3	57.3	45.2	35.8	28.8	27.8
Pakistan	104.6	95.5	86.1	78.4	71.3	62.9	61.2
Sri Lanka	18.1	16.5	13.8	11.7	9.6	7.8	7.5
South Asia	**89.4**	**78.2**	**66.6**	**56.3**	**46.8**	**37.9**	**36.4**

Source Compiled from World Bank database as updated on September 2018

to the world IMR of 29. However, it is clear from the data that the decline is slower in this region as compared to the rest of the world (Table 2.7).

Basic health infrastructure in South Asia is well below the world average. The region suffers from a shortage of physicians as well as hospital beds—on average one physician cares for more than 1600 patients whereas the world average was around 700 per 1600 patients. Additionally, there are only 0.9 hospital beds per 1000 people, compared to 2.9 beds against 1000 people in the world.[21] Conditions in the Maldives

---

[21] This data is for 2010 as updated on September 2018, World Development Indicators.

and Sri Lanka are much better than those found in other countries of the region. The Maldives has even surpassed the world average for these indicators. But the trend in Afghanistan is alarming as the number of doctors has not increased at the same rate of increase for other countries of the region. However, Nepal has significantly improved the availability of doctors at a much faster rate than other nations—in 1990, 1 doctor was caring for around 20,000 patients (0.24 hospital beds per 1000 people) which has improved to around 1 doctor per 1672 people by 2014. Improvement in India and Bangladesh has been consistently positive. Human development indices and indicators as published in 2018 show that on average as a region, South Asia had 7.8 physicians per 10,000 people, which is slightly better than Sub-Saharan Africa which had 1.9 physicians. Europe and Central Asia had the highest number of physicians per 10,000 people at 24.7. The average number of hospital beds per 10,000 people is 58 in high human development countries, compared with 9 in medium human development countries, and 13 in low human development countries (UNDP, 2018, p. 8). Looking at these figures it is clear that South Asia needs significant improvement in healthcare, but it is possible if a greater state priority is placed on health. Further, as explored by India and Bangladesh, private-public partnerships can build better health infrastructure for improvement in the outcome indicators viz-a-viz human well-being. The policies of different governments for improving health infrastructure, indicators, and conditions as a whole are discussed in Chap. 3.

2.5   Trends in Education Indicators

Education has been considered a human right in global policy discussions (Bajaj & Kidwai, 2016) for more than half a century. It is one of the most important factors used to gauge the well-being of a population. Though it was defined as a basic human right in the 1948 Universal Declaration of Human Rights, as adopted by the UN, the South Asian region has witnessed remarkable growth in education just in the preceding two decades. Despite this improvement, the region remains least literate as compared to other regions.

Between 1990 and 2017 the expected years of schooling (number of years of schooling that a child of school-entrance age can expect to receive, if prevailing patterns of age specific enrolment rates persist throughout the child's life) across South Asia have almost doubled, and that is a good sign. On average, Sri Lankans were expected to spend 11.3 years in school (the highest in the region) in 1990 and 11.4 years in 1991, whereas an Afghani was expected to spend merely 2.6 years in school (the lowest in the region) in 1990 and 2.9 years in 1991. Over the last 27 years, most part of the region has made steady progress in education. In 2017, Sri Lanka had the highest expected years of school attendance at 13.9 years, contrasting with Pakistan which averaged only 8.6 years (Fig. 2.12) and was the lowest in the region. Afghanistan has improved schooling years drastically, more so than any other

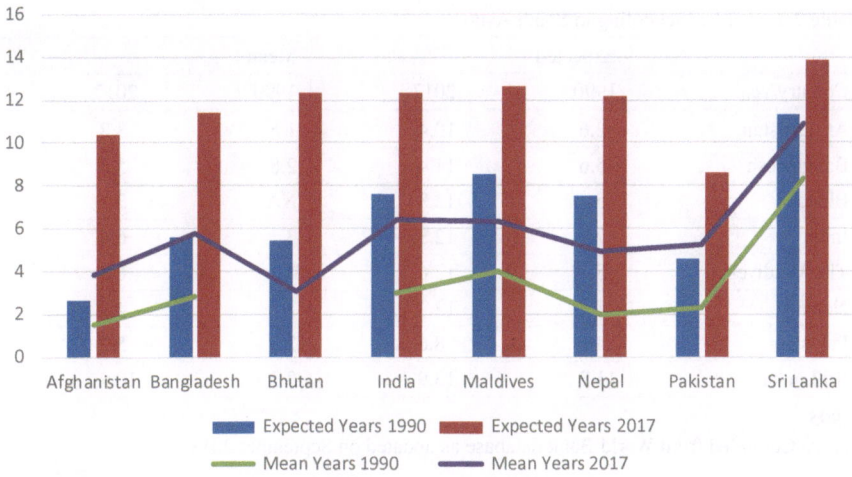

Fig. 2.12 Trends in years of education

country in South Asia as there was a fourfold increase during the 1990–2017 period—followed by Bhutan, Bangladesh, and Pakistan respectively. The region thus shows consistent positive progress in expected average years of school attendance.

On an average, a person of 25 years or more residing in South Asia spent 3.1 years attending school in 1991. This has gone up to 5.8 years in 2017 (Fig. 2.12). Afghanistan, Nepal, and Pakistan have been able to improve these numbers by encouraging more and more children to go to school which is reflected in the mean years of schooling (average number of years of education received by people aged 25 and older, converted from education attainment levels using official durations of each level) data which shows an increase by more than double between 1990 and 2017. These countries previously had the lowest rank in the region in this indicator. India doubled its mean years of schooling during the period as well. Sri Lanka and the Maldives were already far ahead of the other countries of the region in 1991. The data examining years of education and mean years of schooling shows that youth are inclined to seek education and are spending more time compared in school to previous decades (1960–1990) to acquire knowledge and improve their educational level. The governments across the region have made efforts to improve education levels to achieve the "Education for All"[22] target as committed by the SDGs (Table 2.8).

Adult literacy rate (ALR) is one of the important outcomes to assess literacy levels and the effectiveness of efforts by respective governments to improve education levels. ALR is the percentage of the population aged 15 and older that can, with understanding, both read and write a short simple statement on everyday life. The ALR of the South Asian region is slightly better than Sub-Saharan Africa. In 2017, South Asia had an ALR of 68.7% compared to 59.9% in the case of Sub-Saharan Africa. In the rest of the world, Europe and Central Asia as a region had the highest

---

[22]The background of Education for All or EFA program has been discussed in Chap. 3.

Table 2.8 Years of schooling in South Asia

	Expected		Mean	
Country/year	1990	2017	1990	2017
Afghanistan	2.6	10.4	1.5	3.8
Bangladesh	5.6	11.4	2.8	5.8
Bhutan	5.4	12.3	NA	3.1
India	7.6	12.3	3	6.4
The Maldives	8.5[a]	12.6	4	6.3
Nepal	7.5	12.2	2	4.9
Pakistan	4.6	8.6	2.3	5.2
Sri Lanka	11.3	13.9	8.3	10.9

[a]1995

Source Compiled from World Bank database as updated on September 2018

ALR at 98.2% (UNDP, 2018, p. 57). The data of the ALR for the countries in South Asia is scattered and time-series data is not available, yet on the basis of available data if country-wise comparisons of improvements in the region are made, it shows that Afghanistan has the poorest level (31.74% in 2011) whereas the Maldives has the best at more than 98% in 2016. Bangladesh has almost doubled its ALR during 1991–2016 from 35.22 to 72.76%. India, where three-fourths of South Asians reside, had a 69.3% literacy rate in 2011, as compared to Pakistan (which is home to a little more than 10% of the population of South Asia) who had around a 55% literacy rate in 2011 (Fig. 2.13). It will take a few more decades for this region to achieve the goal of "Education for All". Sri Lanka and the Maldives have outperformed the other countries of the region as in case of health parameters. Yet Pakistan, Nepal, and

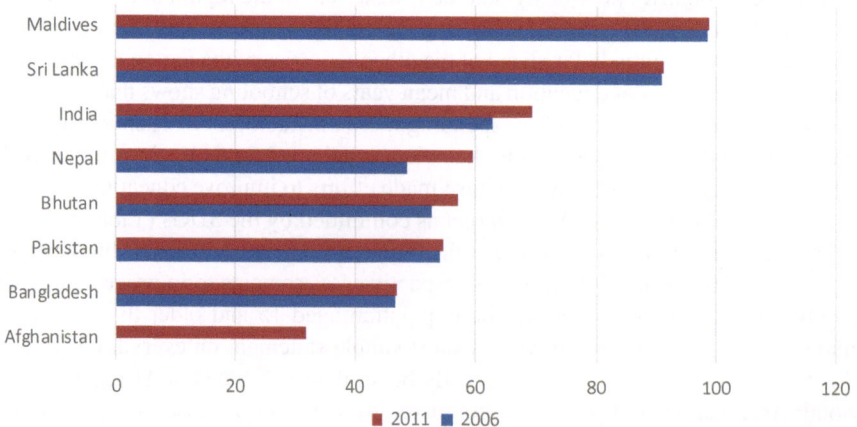

Fig. 2.13 Adult literacy rate in South Asian countries

Bangladesh need to put more effort into eradicating illiteracy. Overall, all the countries of the region have shown improvements in their literacy levels which validates the point that the efforts of the respective governments in the South Asia region are worthwhile. Many programs have been launched to improve overall literacy rates, thereby improving the well-being of citizens which shall be discussed in Chap. 3.

Gender deficits in education are prevalent and wide. On average, 60% of women aged 25 and older have acquired at least some secondary education, compared with 67% of men. This discrepancy is particularly large for the low human development group—15% (women) versus 29% (men). And South Asia has the largest gender gap in education (15 percentage points)[23] with the high percentage referring to educated men.

Bangladesh, after enacting the right to education in its Compulsory Primary Education Act in 1990, has made significant improvements in raising school participation. Compared to 71% in 1980, the gross enrolment rate in primary schools has increased to 100% in 2004 in Bangladesh. However, the primary school completion rate is the lowest in the region at 70% for male students and 80% for female students. Nevertheless, Bangladesh has shown enormous progress in turning around the gender gap in primary and secondary enrolment to the extent that girls' enrolment has exceeded that of boys. By contrast, Nepal has a very recent history of mass education and it has made remarkable progress in increasing access despite political shifts and turmoil that have affected the provision of education (Bajaj & Kidwai, 2016).

The Maldives, despite being a small country, has the highest literacy rate in the region. The ALR for men and women is the same, which indicates an evident unparalleled gender equality. In comparison, girls in Pakistan as well as children of low socioeconomic status or from rural regions continue to have less access to primary education (Dundar, Beteille, Riboud, & Deolalikar, 2014, p. 2). Overall, members of the same gender, especially true for women, are motivated by success stories from other women, and therefore perform better in educational settings. Beaman, Duflo, Pande, and Topalova (2012) found that female students were more highly motivated to succeed when their local administration was led by women. Pakistan and Afghanistan still lag behind the other countries in the region as far as education standards are concerned. It is disheartening to note that education and skill development are among the two most neglected areas of economic development in Pakistan (Amjad et al., 2015). There have been improvements as evidenced by the fact that the number of out-of-school children is going down across the region. The enrolment rates are also on the rise, which is reflected through mean years of schooling.

There is a huge gap between the literacy rates of men and women in Afghanistan as literacy rate for male it was 61.9% whereas for females it was 32.1%.[24] Gender inequality has been recognized as one of the major bottlenecks affecting human well-being. UNDP initiated developing related indices in order to track the status across countries. In that direction Gender-related Development Index (GDI) and Gender

---

[23] See UNDP (2014, p. 40).

[24] See UNDP (2018, p. 56: Table 9).

Table 2.9 HDI and gender inequality index (GII)

SA rank	Country	World rank	World HDI rank	GII values
1	The Maldives	77	101	0.343
2	Sri Lanka	80	76	0.354
3	Bhutan	117	134	0.476
4	Nepal	118	149	0.480
5	India	127	130	0.524
6	Pakistan	133	150	0.541
7	Bangladesh	134	136	0.542
8	Afghanistan	153	168	0.653

Source Compiled with the help of data obtained from UNDP (2018: 38–41)

Empowerment Measure (GEM) were introduced in 1995 to gauge gender development and empowerment status. As most of the indicators were found to be only suitable for developed countries and were closely related to GDP per capita, the indices were questioned. It was in that response that in 2010, Gender Inequality Index (GII) was introduced replacing GDI and GEM. GII is based on five basic indicators bracketed under three dimensions. The dimensions are reproductive health, empowerment, and economic status or labor market participation. These dimensions are measured through maternal mortality ratio and adolescent birth rates for health; proportion of parliamentary seats occupied by females and proportion of adult females and males aged 25 years and older with at least some secondary education for empowerment; and labor force participation rate of female and male populations aged 15 years and older for labor market participation.

GII for 160 countries is available for 2018 which shows that South Asian region is just better than Sub-Saharan Africa and Arab States whereas the Europe and Central Asia has best values. In South Asian region, Afghanistan was ranked lowest at 153 whereas the Maldives was ranked the highest at 77th rank (Table 2.9). When a comparison across the countries of the region between HDI rank and GII rank is done, it is seen that except Sri Lanka in all other countries HDI is higher than GII (Fig. 2.14). India and Bangladesh have closest proximity in the region between GII and HDI, and Nepal has the widest gap. Concerted efforts are required for bridging the gap through appropriate policies and their effective implementation for improving health infrastructure, assuring empowerment through allowing participation of women in politics and labor force. It would strengthen the status of women and gender parity could be maintained.

Although educational well-being in South Asia has improved over the period of 1990–2017, it has not kept pace with gains in the rest of the world. International agencies have made contributions to improve educational outcomes in South Asia, but inherent territorial problems, religious stigmas, gender inequality, and concentration on quantity rather than quality have greatly hindered the cause of educational well-being in the region.

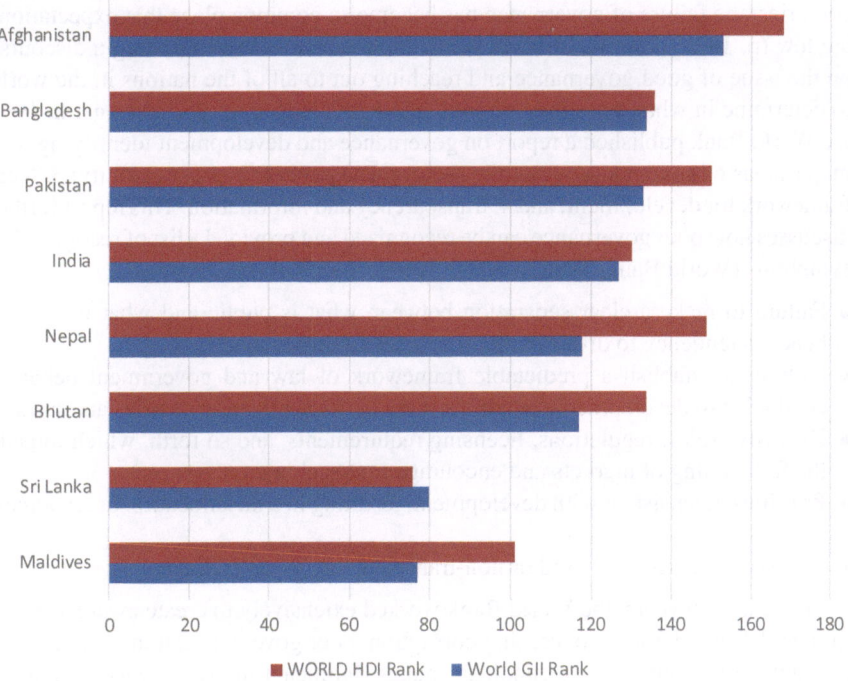

Fig. 2.14 Status in gender inequality index vis-à-vis HDI

2.6 Governance in South Asia

Governance primarily concerns the use of power or authority by the state or government entity for the welfare of its citizens. Broadly, it also includes the management of resources in the interest of the country. In democratic systems, citizens are expected to elect their representatives, forming the government which assures their well-being and effective management of resources. The science of wealth (resources) and welfare (HWB) which relates to acquisition and maintenance of territory is called *Arthashastra* (see Rangarajan, 1992, p. 79). *The Arthashastra* was written by Kautilya, the chief advisor to the first Mauryan emperor Chandragupta, around 320 BC and is considered one of the world's oldest treatises on the economic administration and governance. It talks of acquiring and maintaining resources or wealth, as well as reflections on the welfare of subjects by the ruler.

Today, the World Bank (1992) defines governance as the manner in which power is exercised in the management of a country's economic and social resources for development. Working on a book on Sub-Saharan Africa, a World Bank team published its work in 1989 (World Bank, 1989) where apart from many other concerns such as investing in people, corruption, role of private sector, role of industry, etc., it examined the so-called "crisis' of governance" and found that in many African countries, the failure of governance has become so common place that expectations are low (p. 192). This World Bank publication is credited for initiating a discourse on the issue of good governance and reaching out to all of the nations in the world to determine in what ways they provide good governance to their citizens. In 1992 the World Bank published a report on governance and development identifying four major areas of governance: 1. public sector management; 2. accountability; 3. legal framework for development; and 4. transparency and information. This report further discusses how poor governance can be recognized and provided a list of recognizable symptoms (World Bank, 1992, p. 9):

- Failure to make a clear separation between what is public and what is private, hence, a tendency to divert public resources for private gain;
- Failure to establish a predictable framework of law and government behavior conducive to development, or arbitrariness in the application of rules and laws;
- Excessive rules, regulations, licensing requirements, and so forth, which impede the functioning of markets and encourage rent-seeking;
- Priorities inconsistent with development, resulting in a misallocation of resources; and
- Excessively narrowly based or non-transparent decision making.

In the last 26 years, the World Bank worked extensively to create awareness and initiate debate on issues concerning corruption, poor governance, transparency, and accountability. The use of technology makes significant improvements in creating better systems to assure efficient governance. Reduction in human intervention with the use of technology driven solutions have produced results in a more timely and effective manner. The World Development Report 2017 (World Bank, 2017) focused on governance and examined related facts and figures from across a multitude of worldwide nations which raised awareness and provided cross comparisons. The background paper on this World Development Report, written by Lateef (2016) provides important highlights and the motivation for focusing on governance as a theme of the report.

One can visualize the strong relationship between good governance and HWB which strengthens the trust of citizens in the government so that they are more willing to work towards the nation's well-being. Good governance becomes more important in the countries where income levels are low and income opportunities are in a nascent stage. The South Asian region has been a victim of poor governance. There have been excellent government plans and strategies implemented in South Asia, but at the ground level the benefits do not reach to the intended population. This is compounded by a poor accountability system, which means that often the middlemen who are involved in the process of delivery are not held responsible. Corruption levels are alarming across region. The condition and trends in governance are discussed for having country-wise comparison. The Worldwide Governance Indicators[25] are used as outcome variables for gauging effective governance. There are six aggregate indicators on the basis of these broad dimensions of governance:

---

[25] See Kaufmann, Kraay, and Mastruzzi (2010) for detailed methodology of the indicators.

1. Voice and Accountability: Reflects perceptions of the extent to which a country's citizens are able to participate in selecting their government, as well as freedom of expression, freedom of association, and a free media.
2. Political Stability and Absence of Violence/Terrorism: Political Stability and Absence of Violence/Terrorism measure perceptions of the likelihood of political instability and/or politically-motivated violence, including terrorism.
3. Government Effectiveness: Reflects perceptions of the quality of public services, the quality of the civil service and the degree of its independence from political pressures, the quality of policy formulation and implementation, and the credibility of the government's commitment to such policies.
4. Regulatory Quality: Reflects perceptions of the ability of the government to formulate and implement sound policies and regulations that permit and promote private sector development.
5. Rule of Law: Reflects perceptions of the extent to which agents have confidence in and abide by the rules of society, and in particular the quality of contract enforcement, property rights, the police, and the courts, as well as the likelihood of crime and violence.
6. Control of Corruption: Reflects perceptions of the extent to which public power is exercised for private gain, including both petty and grand forms of corruption, as well as "capture" of the state by elites and private interests.

The percentile rank of South Asian countries among all countries has been taken into consideration for analysis here ranging from 0 (lowest) to 100 (highest), based on the large number of enterprises, citizens, and expert survey respondents in industrial and developing countries. The World Bank Group uses this data to allocate resources across geographies.

Between 1996 and 2017 (Table 2.10), across different nations, it is clear that Afghanistan is the poorest in terms of effective governance. India has the most vibrant democracy in the region, which is reflected through its rank in voice and accountability, as it ranked first in the region in 1996 as well as in 2017 (Fig. 2.15). When examining the changes in rank during 1996–2017, Bhutan has improved its

Table 2.10 Worldwide governance indicators rank (aggregate)

Country/year	1996	2000	2006	2011	2016	2017
Afghanistan	1.8	1.6	5.3	3.9	8.0	7.9
Bangladesh	26.6	25.3	17.4	22.4	22.7	21.8
Bhutan	55.1	56.4	57.0	54.3	64.1	68.6
India	44.6	46.4	46.7	42.6	45.7	46.3
The Maldives	60.9	59.0	49.6	39.1	38.1	34.4
Nepal	42.6	33.4	23.3	21.3	23.5	26.2
Pakistan	24.3	20.9	24.6	18.6	20.4	22.9
Sri Lanka	44.4	44.6	41.9	41.8	49.5	46.8

Source Compiled values from the given data of each component of WGI

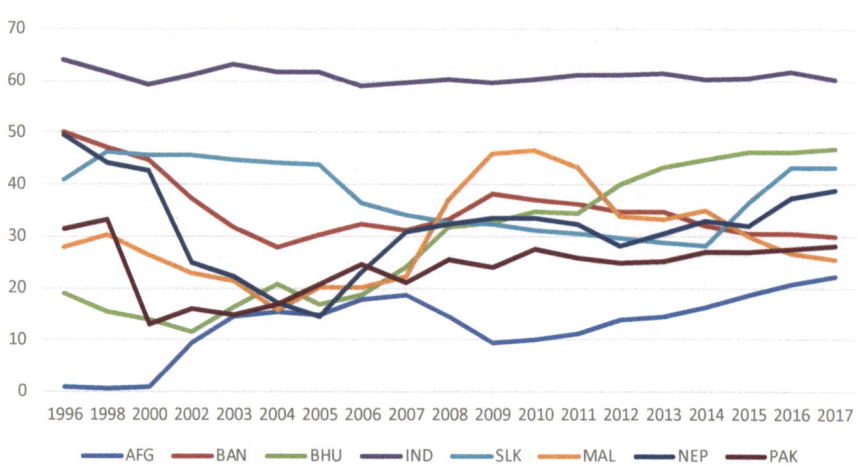

Fig. 2.15 Governance: voice and accountability

rank which is to be expected as it had its first general elections in 2008—marking the commencement of constitutional democracy. Conditions in Bangladesh and Nepal have gotten worse during this period. When the ranks of the last ten years are examined, Sri Lanka has improved its position much more so than other countries (except Bhutan) which reflects its improved handling of problems through decentralization affecting people's perception in general.

When national rankings are awarded on the basis of political stability and absence of violence and terrorism (Fig. 2.16), the statistics show that conditions in Afghanistan and Pakistan have worsened over time. The Maldives enjoyed the highest rank among South Asian countries in 1996, followed by Bhutan. It had strong

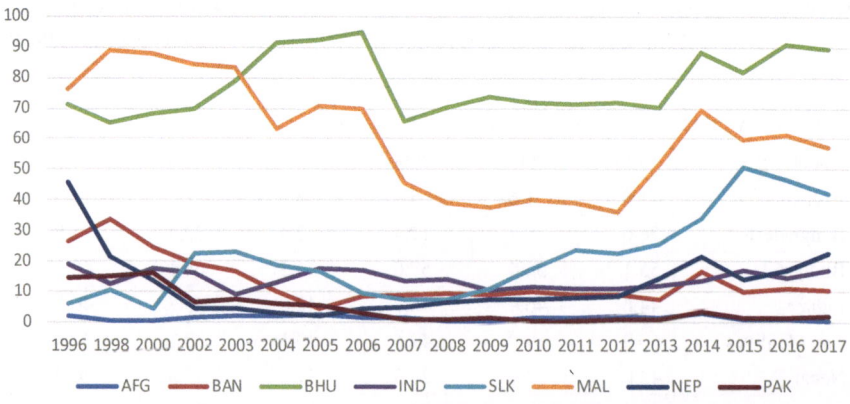

Fig. 2.16 Governance: political stability and no violence

democratic leader in Maumoon Abdul Gayoom, who won the 1993 elections—winning 92% of the votes casted—and he again proved his prowess in 1998. He provided strong leadership between 1978 and 2008, which is reflected through data collected on the Maldives political stability. Barring few incidences, the Maldives was peaceful until 2008. Bhutan has been the most peaceful and politically stable country among all the South Asian nations, as it ranked first in terms of political stability among all countries of the region in 2017. Conditions in Bangladesh and Nepal have not been very stable, but Sri Lanka has consistently improved in terms of their political stability. India has been at roughly the same position across the period and has maintained its rank within the region (5th in 1996 as well as in 2017).

If one examines these rankings in terms of the size of a nation, the data makes a case that small nations are managed much more effectively than large nations. Bhutan and the Maldives (two least populated countries of the region) perform best whereas India, Pakistan, and Bangladesh (three most populated countries of the region) perform worst on this indicator. Excepting Bhutan, the whole region has experienced political instability paired with violence and has suffered from terrorism-both from within as well as from outside.

The third indicator is very important as it tracks government's effectiveness based on the quality of services and independence from political pressures, in addition to examining its commitment towards well-being of its citizens. There is visible improvement in this indicator in the case of Afghanistan, though the nation still remains the lowest ranked between 1996 and 2017 (Fig. 2.17). The government of Bhutan has been consistently most effective in the region over last two decades. Though the Maldives had a stable government when first ranked in 1996, it has failed to maintain that stability. In 2017, both Bhutan and India have surpassed the Maldives. The conditions in India have marginally improved. The governments of Nepal, Bangladesh, and Pakistan have not been able to maintain their effectiveness which is reflected through the rankings.

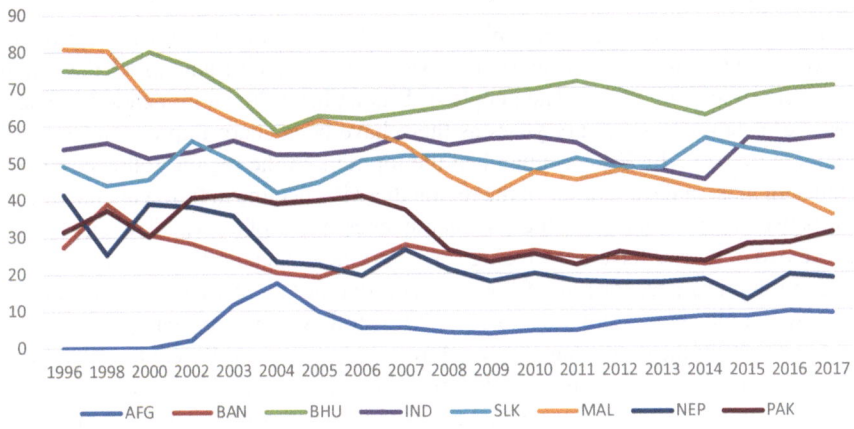

Fig. 2.17 Governance: government effectiveness

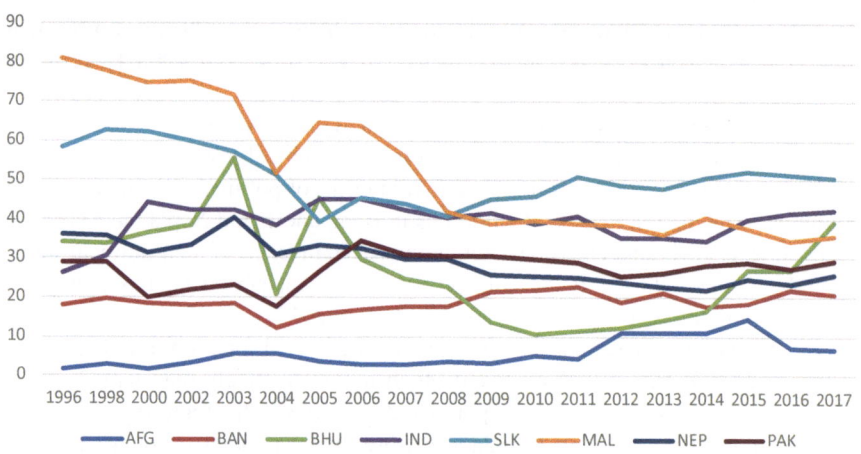

Fig. 2.18 Governance: regulatory quality

In terms of a sound and effective regulatory system, conditions in the Maldives have worsened over the years (Fig. 2.18). Bhutan has experienced fluctuations across the years as it was in a transitory phase from a monarchial system to democratic structure. India, between 1996 and 2017, witnessed the introduction of several landmark regulations by the government—such as Right To Information (RTI) and Right To Education (RTE)—resulting in improved general governance and improvement on accountability measures. This has almost definitely created a positive perception in the minds of the Indian people. To support this, the indicator on regulatory quality shows an uptrend for India. Pakistan has also been able to improve its position, but conditions in Nepal have worsened. Bangladesh and Afghanistan have shown only marginal improvements, but not as good as of other nations of the region. They must formulate better policies for their respective countries in order to cater to the needs of their citizens.

The trends concerning maintaining rule of law in India has not been positive between 1996 and 2017, but in 1996 it was ranked the best among all the South Asian countries (Fig. 2.19). The people of Bhutan have shown tremendous respect for rule of law in last twenty years as there have been sharp improvements in its comparative rank. In 2017, Bhutan had the top rank in the region, followed by Sri Lanka. In most of the countries of the region there is a decline in following the rule of law between 1996 and 2017, which is much steeper in case of the Maldives and Nepal. These two countries have been facing severe political instability, affecting people's perception on respect for rule of law. As seen in other indicators, Afghanistan had the lowest rank across between 1996 and 2017, followed by Pakistan.

Most parts of the region have suffered from corruption of different kinds and volume. Opening of economy through liberalization and privatization in 1991 has provided significant opportunities resulting in economic growth, but it has also increased the incidences of corruption, at policy level as well as on implementation level. The

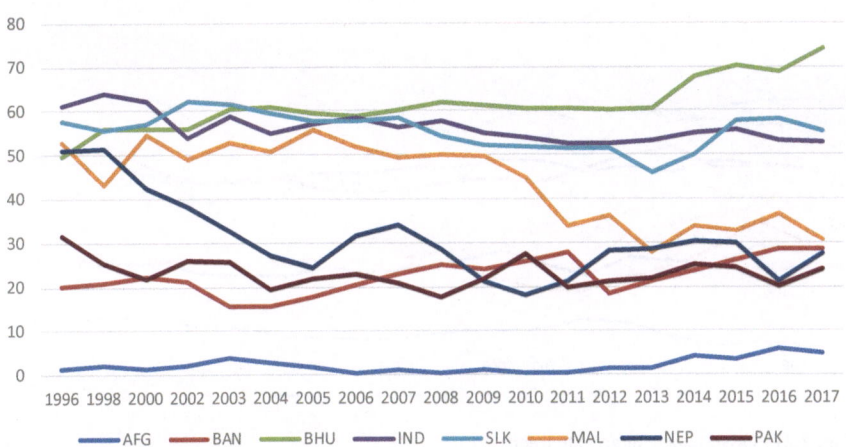

Fig. 2.19 Governance: rule of law

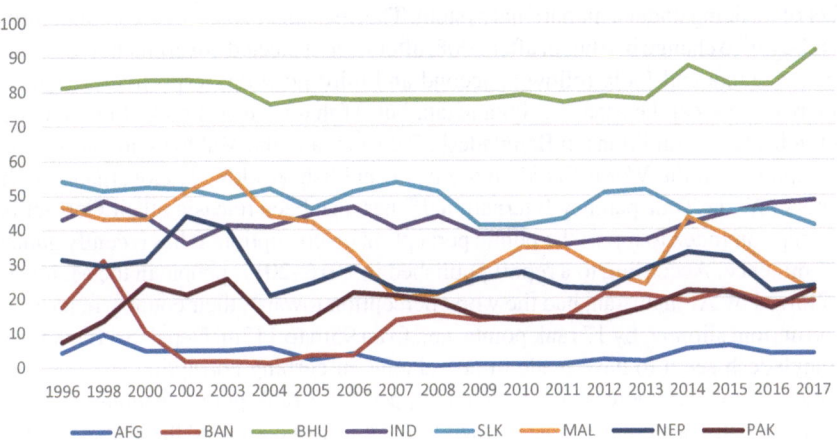

Fig. 2.20 Governance: control of corruption

perception of Indian population is negatively affected because of poor governance (Das, 2012). Bhutan has been an exception in controlling corruption as it maintained a substantial lead over other countries in the region consistently between 1996 and 2017 (Fig. 2.20). Conditions in Afghanistan are ominous. Bangladesh, the Maldives, Nepal, and Pakistan have similar positions in terms of the control of corruption, but all of these are better than Afghanistan. Though India ranked fourth in 1996, it has risen to second place in 2017 which reflects its strong commitment to eliminate corruption. India's policies are drafted and implemented in a highly transparent manner showing an improvement over their earlier practices.

When overall Worldwide Governance Indicators (Fig. 2.21) are put together and the average of their rank percentile is taken (Table 2.10), Bhutan is revealed to have

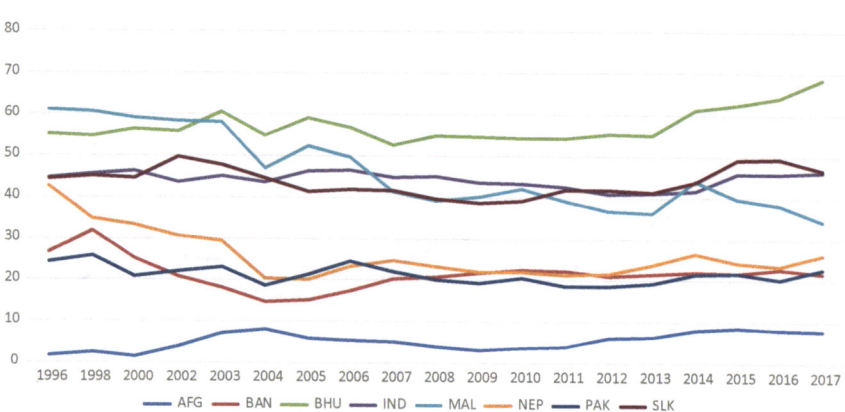

Fig. 2.21 Governance: aggregate trends

the best rank across all indicators except Voice and Accountability—mainly due to the fact of its being under a monarchial system. This measure (Voice and Accountability) has begun to change in Bhutan after 2008, after its first elected government was sworn in. Sri Lanka and India follow in second and third position, respectively. Signs of improvement can be seen in Afghanistan, but Afghanistan still ranks lowest across all indicators. Conditions in Bangladesh, Pakistan, and the Maldives are worsening.

Apart from the World Bank's initiative to publish Worldwide Governance Indicators (WGI), Transparency International[26] has also been releasing their Corruption Perception Index to report the public perception on corruption. It has recently gained prominence. According to a report published in 2016–2017, people in the Maldives, followed by Afghanistan, had the worst perception towards their country in terms of corruption, slipping by 17 rank points, i.e., from 95th to 112th. Nepal, Sri Lanka, and Bangladesh seem to have made improvements in curbing corruption as their comparative rankings increased. But India slipped by 2 rank points. Among all South Asian countries, Bhutan has performed the best as its people had the best perception as compared to other countries in the region. If the rank positions are compared among countries in the region, Bhutan is the best followed by India, Sri Lanka, and the Maldives. These perceptions agree with the Worldwide Governance Indicators as discussed earlier.

On governance, the South Asian region has much larger challenge to respond. The countries have to put in place a better system, build trust and maintain better law and order. All the countries of the region need to focus on governance in order to improve HWB. Political will and determination to deal with terrorist activities would boost the morale of citizens, which will be reflected positively in future governance outcomes.

---

[26]The information is based on the Corruption Perception Index 2017 retrieved from: https://www.transparency.org/news/feature/corruption_perceptions_index_2017.

2.7 Subjective Well-Being and Happiness

Policymakers from Britain to Bhutan have increasingly turned to subjective well-being (SWB)— also referred to as happiness or life satisfaction—to complement traditional measures of economic performance such as GDP and unemployment (Burchardt, 2013). SWB is used as a proxy for quality of life (QOL), happiness, and well-being. Determination of QOL is based on the premise that once human needs are fulfilled, SWB will steadily increase and, in turn, will be expressed as a positive attitude that can be measured using standardized SWB tools (Costanza et al., 2007). SWB refers to how people experience the quality of their lives and includes both emotional reactions and cognitive judgments. The best way to assess a person's life satisfaction is to ask the person directly. It reduces the possibility of manipulation; however, at the same time it is a limited assessment method as it represents the individual's response at a specific point in time. However, it is considered the best way to obtain a firsthand opinion of a person's level of satisfaction with different variables. "Assessing the appraisal of life in a nation requires that the total of experienced well-being is estimated. This sum of experience is denoted by the concept of "happiness." Happiness is a person's overall evaluation of his/her life as-a-whole" (Veenhoven, 1996). Different agencies and individuals have conducted surveys using suitable tools to track the status of life satisfaction (or happiness) across world regions.

SWB data for the South Asia region is not consistently available in a uniform format, making comparisons difficult. However, some data can be obtained through the World Database of Happiness, the WVS, and the Gallup opinion poll. The data from the World Happiness Reports have also been used since their first publication.

In 1984, Ruut Veenhoven published his book titled *Conditions of Happiness*[27] based on his doctoral work entitled "Factors of influence on happiness." The work involved empirical investigation to validate the indicators of happiness based on 245 studies, resulting in over 4000 observations. The full details were published as *Databook of Happiness*.[28] This work was the impetus for the development of the World Database of Happiness (WDH), which is perhaps the most robust archival database on happiness freely available and hosted by the Erasmus University Rotterdam, The Netherlands. The WDH gauges life satisfaction using the Cantril Ladder: "Suppose the top of the ladder represents the best possible life for you and the bottom of the ladder the worst possible life, where on this ladder do you feel you personally stand at the present time".[29] It is 10 step ladder indicating that if one is at step 1, it is the worst possible life and if one is at step 10 it is the best possible life for him/her. The ladder as devised by Cantril (1965) is based on the study of hope, fear, and happiness of persons in 14 countries around the world and is one of the most widely used tools to develop scales on human perception. It was primarily a self-anchoring striving scale where a person was asked about their own assumptions, perceptions,

---

[27] See Veenhoven (1984a).

[28] See Veenhoven (1984b).

[29] This is an adaptation used by Ruut Veenhoven, given in the Exhibit 4/1a at page 67 of Veenhoven (1984a).

goals, and values and the respondents were to choose a place on the ladder at that given point of time. For happiness and well-being research it was found to be more appropriate as compared to other scales.

The perception of people is tracked through using Cantril ladder which is compiled for different nations. The database provides a consolidated figure of life satisfaction for South Asia in 2011 at 4.94[30] (on the scale of 1–10). Except for the Maldives, data for all other countries in the South Asian region is available for the 2005–2014 period, which has been compiled (Table 2.11) and compared with the values present between 2000 and 2009. For 2000–2009, only scattered data was available for Bangladesh, India, Nepal, Pakistan, and India. People in India had a higher level of life satisfaction (5.5) than those in other South Asian countries between 2000 and 2009, which was maintained at the same level for 2005–2014 as well (Fig. 2.22). However, during between 2005 and 2014, Pakistan had the highest life satisfaction (6) and Afghanistan had the lowest levels of life satisfaction in South Asia.

Happy life years, a product of life expectancy and life satisfaction, provide a closer look at the relationship between these objective and subjective measures (Veenhoven, 1996). The happy life years score could be a better measure for studying health well-being because it goes beyond life expectancy and considers subjective measures that are based on people's own perceptions. Between 2000 and 2009, Sri Lanka had the highest (36.2 years) level of average happy life years and Pakistan had the lowest (32.5 years). For the period between 2005 and 2014, happy life years measured 41 years (highest in the region) for Bhutan and at 25.2 years for Afghanistan, which is incidentally the lowest in the region.

The World Values Survey (WVS) provides data (Table 2.12) on life satisfaction (or, in some waves, satisfaction with life). India was included in five of the six waves[31] of data collected between 1990 and 2014. The data for Bangladesh and Pakistan is

Table 2.11 Life satisfaction (LS) and happy life years (HLY)

Countries	2000–09		2005–14	
	LS mean	HLY	LS mean	HLY
Afghanistan	NA	NA	4.1	25.2
Bangladesh	5.3	33.3	5.3	37.1
Bhutan	NA	NA	5.6	41
India	5.5	35.1	5.5	36.6
Nepal	5.3	33.3	5.3	36.4
Pakistan	5	32.5	6	40.1
Sri Lanka	5.1	36.2	5.1	37.6

Source Compiled from World Database of Happiness data of different countries

[30] See R. Veenhoven, *Distributional findings on Happiness in Multiple nations (ZZ), region South Asia*, World Database of Happiness, Erasmus University Rotterdam, The Netherlands. Accessed on 2018-02-06 at http://worlddatabaseofhappiness.eur.nl.

[31] The waves are the intervals of collection of data on life satisfaction as reflected in Fig. 2.23.

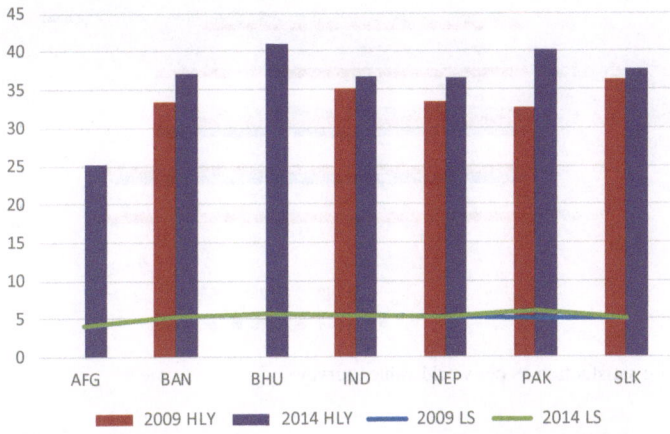

Fig. 2.22 Life satisfaction and happy life years as per world database of happiness

Table 2.12 Life satisfaction mean values—WVS

WVS wave	Year	Bangladesh	India	Pakistan
II	1990–1994	NA	6.7	NA
III	1995–1998	6.41	6.53	NA
IV	2000–2004	5.78	5.14	4.85
V	2005–2009	NA	5.8	NA
VI	2010–2014	NA	5.08	7.54

Source Compiled from World Values Survey data on different waves

available only in two waves (fourth and sixth waves; and third and fourth waves, respectively). The WVS does not provide data for other countries of South Asia. The latest wave for which data is available is sixth wave (2010–2014). The respondents are asked to reply on a 10-point scale (1 being dissatisfied and 10 being satisfied) to the question, "All things considered, how much satisfied are you with your life as a whole these days?" The seventh wave responses are in process and these are going to be available online by mid-2020.[32] When we look at the latest available WVS data over time, we see a downward trend in Bangladesh and India, and an upward trend in Pakistan (Fig. 2.23). Considering the internal problems that Pakistan has experienced in the last 5 years, it is difficult to believe that the residents have experienced such a high level of life satisfaction.

Owing to the small number of respondents for these surveys (e.g., Wave VI, 1591 for India and 1200 for Pakistan) and the scattered nature of the data, it is difficult to be convinced that these surveys reflect the correct SWB of the people of the region. Also, because SWB responses are subjective and reflect the respondent's feelings only at a

---

[32]This information is taken from the website of the World Values Survey http://www.worldvaluessurvey.org/WVSContents.jsp.

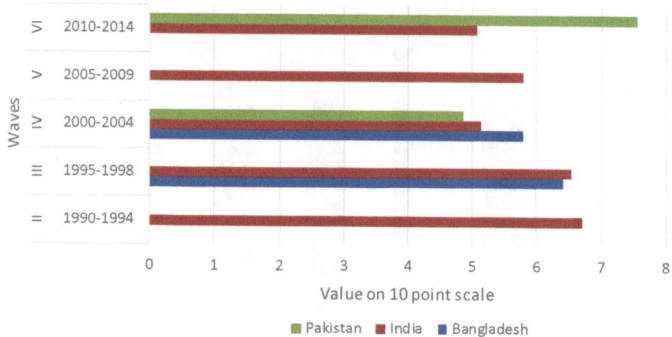

Fig. 2.23 Life satisfaction as per world values survey

specific moment in time, it is difficult to believe that they provide an accurate holistic picture. Between 2007 and 2011, the number of people who reported that they were "very happy" increased 2% globally; however, for India this response increased by 5%. In this study, India was the only country representing South Asia (Wright, 2012).

In April 2012, Jigme Y. Thinley, the then Prime Minister of Bhutan, was invited by the United Nations to host the first high level meeting, calling happiness scholars from across the world to discuss measuring happiness. It was the first time when the UN had taken such an initiative for engaging with the happiness scholars and policy makers to deliberate on happiness at international level. The first World Happiness Report (WHR) was released just before this meeting on April 1, 2012, providing foundational text for discussion. This report provided a basis for designing public policies to improve HWB and measuring happiness across nations. It contained a compilation of different works which prioritized 'happiness' in policy discourse rather than 'economic growth'. The case of Bhutan, including its development philosophy of Gross National Happiness (GNH)[33] and its implementation at policy level by the government was discussed at length in this report. The report drew the attention of international media, policymakers, scholars, and happiness enthusiasts. With the exception of the year 2014, the WHR is being published every year providing the ranks of the countries on happiness. The reports are based on the data through the Gallup World Poll. Here (Table 2.13) the ranks of the countries in the South Asian region as given in these reports are discussed as they are consistent and comparable.

The rankings in the GWP, as reflected in the World Happiness Reports, are based on healthy life expectancy, GDP per capita, social support, freedom to make life choices, perception of corruption, education, and generosity. It covers almost all domains of HWB but since it is based on a small sample of the population, its

---

[33] It is important to mention here that it was this tiny kingdom which had voiced its concern for the happiness of its citizens over gross domestic product in the UN session of 1972. Ever since it has been following this philosophy, amid criticism from different corners, on its only philosophical value and not on measurement. It was in 2010 that Bhutan went ahead with measuring GNH and published its report. In 2015, Bhutan published another report on perception of GNH. Detailed version on GNH in Bhutan is provided in Chap. 4.

Table 2.13 Score and ranks in world happiness report (2013–2018)

Country	2013 GWP 2010–12		2015 GWP 2012–14		2016 GWP 2013–15		2017 GWP 2014–16		2018 GWP 2015–17	
	Score	Rank	Score	Rank	Score	Rank	Score	Rank	Score	Rank
Afghanistan	4.040	143	3.575	153	3.360	154	3.794	141	3.632	145
Bangladesh	4.804	108	4.694	109	4.635	110	4.608	110	4.500	115
Bhutan	NA	NA	5.253	79	5.196	84	5.041	97	5.082	97
India	4.772	111	4.565	117	4.404	118	4.315	122	4.190	133
Nepal	4.156	135	4.514	121	4.793	107	4.962	99	4.880	101
Pakistan	5.292	81	5.194	91	5.132	92	5.269	80	5.472	75
Sri Lanka	4.151	137	4.271	132	4.415	117	4.440	120	4.471	116
Number of countries covered	156		158		157		155		156	

Source Compiled from world happiness reports of different years

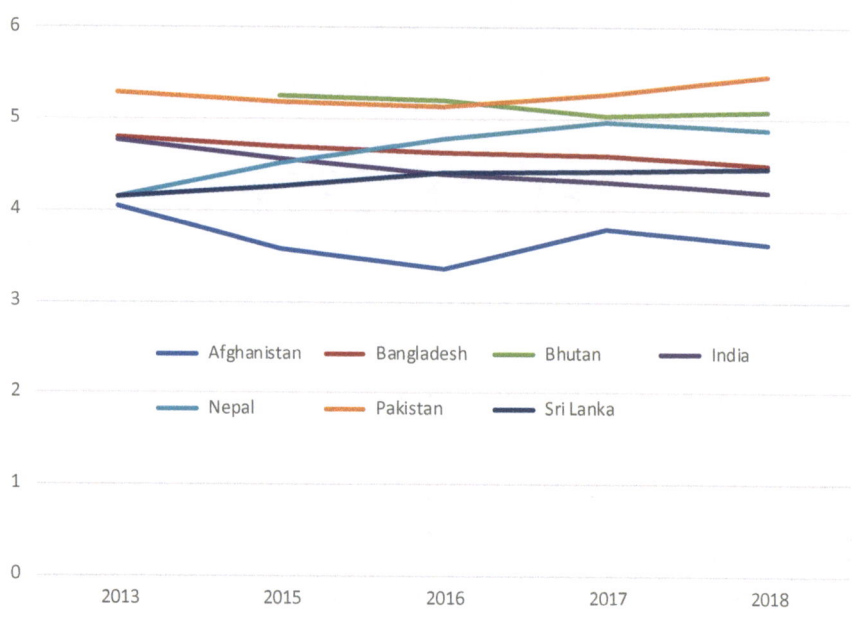

Fig. 2.24 Happiness scores (world gallup poll—world happiness report)

acceptability as such is difficult to admit. The reports do not include the Maldives. It is visible through the reports across years (2013–2018) that Pakistan and Bhutan are among the top two countries in terms of happiness and Afghanistan is at the bottom among all the South Asian countries (Fig. 2.24). The reporting of SWB data from South Asia has been highly inconsistent both in terms of trends over time and concerning the countries represented. However, the GWP has tried to bridge that gap. The sample size used in this poll is very small and does not represent the wide diversity prevalent in all parts of the region. GWP data has many limitations however in the absence of any other consistent data on happiness, this provides some trends.

2.8   Conclusion

The objective of this chapter was to identify and discuss outcome indicators which lead to general HWB. In that direction, data sources from the World Development Indicators, Human Development Report, Worldwide Governance Indicators, Transparency International, World Happiness Report, etc. were used to understand the status of each South Asian country individually as well as of the region as a whole. Wherever possible, comparison with other groups of nations and other regions was also made to get better picture of the world. As more than 25% of the world population lives in the South Asian region, it needs to formulate better policy directions so that the living standards of residents are improved. This would largely be accomplished by enabling them to seek and hold gainful employment. As compared to the other world regions, South Asia trails behind and performs poorly on social indicators like health and education, which are necessities for HWB. It is a commonly held belief that people with limited core capabilities, such as in areas like education and health, are less able to live lives they value.[34] Though health and education are the basics, good governance is also a very important component for building trust, and all these three components strengthen enabling social infrastructure. Empowerment through education makes citizens aware and competent to use their choices, good health assures their better physical well-being, and good governance confirms citizen's loyalty with the government. The very first published issue of the Human Development Report made it very clear that though there is a requirement to focus the policy on the social sector, e.g., human development, the importance of income cannot be ignored and nations must put in place policies to improve industry and trade so that income levels are improved.

The outcome indicators discussed in this chapter show that there have been improvements in most of the sectors examined and that the region is working to strengthen its systems so that governance can be improved. Adoption of technology across the region is important as on one side it facilitates proper delivery of services to citizens and on the other side makes the people involved in the delivery process accountable. Individual capabilities are being enhanced by different kind of policies depending on the specific nation and its priorities. Income levels have improved a lot almost in all countries of the region. The conditions constituting life satisfaction or SWB are not very promising across South Asia currently. The most recent World Happiness Report published reveals that this region lags far behind as most of the countries are ranked below the top hundred countries of the world. Pakistan (75) and Bhutan (97) are the only two countries which are ranked in top 100 countries on the World Happiness Report 2018.

In the following Chap. 3, the input variables shall be discussed so that a clear picture between input and outcome will emerge and the gaps can be identified for better policy focus in the future, which is one of the core objectives of this work.

References

Amjad, R., Chandrasiri, S., Nathan, D., Raihan, S., Verick, S., & Yusuf, A. (2015). What holds back manufacturing in South Asia. *Economic and Political Weekly, 50*(10), 36–45.

Bajaj, M., & Kidwai, H. (2016). Human rights and education policy in South Asia. In K. Mundy, A. Green, R. Lingard, & A. Verger (Eds.), *Handbook of global education policy* (pp. 206–223). Hoboken, NJ: Wiley-Blackwell.

Beaman, L., Duflo, E., Pande, R., & Topalova, P. (2012). Female leadership raises aspirations and educational attainment for girls: A policy experiment in India. *Science, 335*(6068), 582–586.

---

[34]See UNDP (2014: 55).

Burchardt, T. (2013). Should measures of subjective well-being inform policy priorities? *Journal of Poverty and Social Justice, 21*(1), 3–5.

Cantril, H. (1965). *The pattern of human concerns.* New Brunswick, NJ: Rutgers University Press.

Costanza, R., Fisher, B., Ali, A., Beer, C., Bond, L., Boumans, R., et al. (2007). Quality of life: An approach integrating opportunities, human needs, and subjective well-being. *Ecological Economics, 61,* 267–276.

Das, G. (2012). *India grows at night—A liberal case for a strong state.* India: Penguin Books.

Dundar, H., Béteille, T., Riboud, M., & Deolalikar, A. (2014). *Student learning in South Asia: Challenges, opportunities, and policy priorities.* Washington, DC: International Bank for Reconstruction and Development/The World Bank.

Guillen-Royo, M. (2014). Human needs. In A. C. Michalos (Ed.), *Encyclopedia of quality of life and well-being research* (pp. 3027–3030). Dordrecht: Springer Reference.

Haq, M. (1996). *Reflections on human development.* New York: Oxford University Press.

ILO. (2018). *World employment social outlook—Trends 2018.* Geneva, Switzerland: International Labor Organization. Accessed from https://www.ilo.org/wcmsp5/groups/public/—dgreports/—dcomm/—publ/documents/publication/wcms_615594.pdf.

Kaufmann, D., Kraay, A., & Mastruzzi, M. (2010, September 10). *The worldwide governance indicators: Methodology and analytical issues.* Working Paper No. 5430. World Bank Policy Research. Accessed from https://papers.ssrn.com/sol3/papers.cfm?abstract_id=1682130.

Kuznets, S. (1934). *National income, 1929–32, 1934.* New York: National Bureau of Economic Research. Accessed from http://www.nber.org/chapters/c2258.pdf on September 30, 2017.

Lateef, K. S. (2016). *Evolution of the World Bank's thinking on governance.* Background Paper World Development Report 2017—Governance and the Law. Accessed from http://pubdocs.worldbank.org/en/433301485539630301/WDR17-BP-Evolution-of-WB-Thinking-on-Governance.pdf.

OPHI. (2018). *Global multidimensional poverty index 2018: The most detailed picture to date of the world's poorest people.* Oxford, UK: Oxford Poverty and Human Development Initiative, University of Oxford.

Phillips, D. (2006). *Quality of life: Concept, policy and practice.* New York: Routledge.

Rajaram, M. (2009). *Thirukkural—Pearls of inspiration.* New Delhi, India: Rupa Publications.

Ram, R. (1998). Forty years of life span revolution: An exploration of the roles of convergence income and policy. *Economic Development and Cultural Change, 46*(4), 849–857.

Rangarajan, L. N. (Ed.). (1992). *Kautilya—The Arthashastra.* Gurgaon, India: Penguin Random House.

Sirgy, M. J., Lee, D.-J., Miller, C., & Littlefield, J. E. (2004). The impact of globalization on a country's quality of life: Toward an integrated model. *Social Indicators Research, 68*(3), 251–298.

Tiberius, V. (2014). Philosophical theories of well-being. In A. C. Michalos (Ed.), *Encyclopedia of quality of life and well-being research* (pp. 7110–7113). Dordrecht: Springer Reference.

Tsai, M.-C. (2006). Does globalization affect human well-being? *Social Indicators Research, 81,* 103–126.

UNDP. (1990). *Human development report 1990: Concept and measurement of human development, United Nations development program.* New York: Oxford University Press.

UNDP. (2014). *Human development report 2014: Sustaining human progress: Reducing vulnerability and building resilience.* New York: United Nations Development Program.

UNDP. (2018). *Human development indices and indicators 2018 statistical update.* New York: United Nations Development Program.

Vaarama, M., & Pieper, R. (2014). Quality of life and quality of care: An integrated model. In A. C. Michalos (Ed.), *Encyclopedia of quality of life and well-being research* (pp. 5269–5276). Dordrecht: Springer Reference.

Veenhoven, R. (1984a). *Conditions of happiness.* Boston: D. Reidel Publishing.

Veenhoven, R. (1984b). *Data book of happiness: A complementary reference work to 'Conditions of happiness'.* Boston: D. Reidel Publishing.

Veenhoven, R. (1996). Happy life-expectancy: A comprehensive measure of quality-of-life in nations. *Social Indicators Research, 39,* 1–58.

Wagle, U. R., & Koirala, B. (2014). Welfare economics. In A. C. Michalos (Ed.), *Encyclopedia of quality of life and well-being research* (pp. 7029–7032). Dordrecht: Springer Reference.

World Bank. (1989). *Sub-Saharan Africa: From crisis to sustainable growth—A long term perspective study.* Washington DC: The International Bank for Reconstruction and Development, World Bank. http://documents.worldbank.org/curated/en/498241468742846138/pdf/multi0page.pd.

World Bank. (1992). *Governance and development.* Washington DC: The International Bank for Reconstruction and Development, World Bank.

World Bank. (2013). *World development report 2014: Risk and opportunity—Managing risk for development.* Washington, DC: World Bank.

World Bank. (2017). *World development report 2017—Governance and the law..* Washington, DC: The International Bank for Reconstruction and Development, World Bank.

Wright, J. (2012, August 18). *Despite woes, conflicts, world a happier place than in 2007 as 22% (+2 points) of global citizens say they're 'very happy.'* [Ipsos press release]. Retrieved from: https://www.ipsos.com/en-us/despite-woes-conflicts-world-happier-place-2007-22-2-points-global-citizens-say-theyre-very-happy. Accessed on August 18, 2015.

Chapter 3
Major Policy Interventions for Human Well-Being in South Asia

This physical world has no two things alike.
Every comparison is awkwardly rough.
You can put a lion next to a man,
but the placing is hazardous to both.
[Rumi][a]

Abstract This chapter discusses major policy interventions implemented by the respective states and major international non-governmental organizations to promote quality of life and well-being for the people of South Asia. These substantial efforts are continuing into the present era with considerable levels of success. Taken together, these multilateral initiatives are strengthening the region's economic progress and development, especially with respect to both national per capita and GDP. Both outcomes have significant poverty implications in world regions that have historically been characterized by alarmingly high levels of financial poverty and human deprivation. GDP share spent on education and health by each country of the region and its trend over time is discussed for comparison purpose. Major initiatives taken to improve education and health standards by South Asian governments, international agencies, and NGOs are reported to gain a better understanding of regional priorities. The steps proposed and followed in order to combat corruption and the methods designed to deal with governance deficit are examined to hopefully influence future policy direction.

Keywords Human well-being · South Asia · Public policy · Economic well-being · Education well-being · Health well-being · Governance

3.1 Introduction

The state is responsible for the management of national resources and the well-being of its citizens. The citizens in return expect their concerns to be addressed by elected political officials in whom they bestow their trust and assign responsibility to rule. This is the expectation in a democratic system. The governments of South

---

[a]see Banks 1995, p. 177.

© Springer Nature Switzerland AG 2020

V. K. Shrotryia, *Human Well-Being and Policy in South Asia*, Human Well-Being Research and Policy Making, https://doi.org/10.1007/978-3-030-33270-9_3

Asian states work to win the confidence of their people by first identifying the public areas of concern and then by formulating appropriate and executable strategies in order to address these concerns. There must be provisions for investment in human capital through effective systems of health and education, which enable individuals to contribute to the national well-being. The citizens of a country form the base of all development initiatives. Development initiatives are arguably more important for developing and/or poor regions, as those regions lack resources and the allied ability to exploit them. Investments in human capital are of greater importance for developing and/or poor regions for the same reasons.

Primarily, in order to invest in people, the states need to have a strong capital base which is acquired through developing capabilities and competencies to produce and serve. Tax revenue and philanthropies also help states to build capacities to look after the well-being of citizens. Economic growth needs to be translated through greater investment in social development, otherwise it does not serve the purpose of assuring HWB. "Since the mid-20th century, the ultimate aim of government policy in the economic sphere has been sustained growth in GDP and productivity" (Sgroi, Hills, O'Donnell, Oswald, & Proto, 2017, p. 6). This mindset promoted the idea that only wealth or income is important and is further one of the primary reasons why development agencies and individuals started thinking of alternative approaches to measure progress.

As mentioned in the preceding chapter, the South Asian region is rich in diversity and resources but poor in areas such as efficiency, good governance, and social indicators (primarily health and education). The major cause of this stagnation lies in poor social infrastructure and poor governance. Except Afghanistan, Bhutan, Nepal and the Maldives, which comprise little less than 5% population of the region, most of the territories of the region (India, Pakistan, and Bangladesh having more than 95% population in the region) have been under British rule which has affected their resources negatively, and it is just about 70 years that it has tried to improve its development outcomes and indicators enabling it to progress better and compete with countries of the other regional groups. The problems lie not merely with the legacies of colonization, but also with the colonial mindset which has caused significant harm through its feudal policies and influenced the policies negatively.

The outcomes that were discussed in the previous chapter are connected with concerned inputs through policy initiatives and strategies to improve income, education, health, and governance, and to reduce poverty, unemployment, etc. This chapter discusses policy initiatives taken by South Asian governments in last three decades. Policies concerning income (or GDP), health, and education as introduced by respective governments are discussed. General policies resulting in improvement to the governance mechanism are highlighted. As subjective well-being is an outcome variable for which directly policies are not made, there is no related discussion.

The purpose of this book is to examine and deliberate on HWB outcomes and relate them with concerned policy from the prism of well-being (happiness), as that is considered to be the ultimate goal of human life. Measuring economic progress and articulating whether such progress has resulted in making individuals happy, falls under the domain of this work. For that intent, this chapter examines policy initiatives accordingly.

3.2 Policy on Economic Growth and Development

Over the past 70 years, the focus of most of the South Asian governments (India, Sri Lanka, Pakistan, and Bangladesh) has been to first sustain and then to boost the economy by implementing relevant policies. In the initial years, these countries invested their capital in industry and agriculture production. The industries in most South Asian countries were heavily reliant on human labor, as labor is something that the entire region has always been rich in. However, mostly these investments were not significant enough to boost the economies, and they have been conservative in attracting foreign investment. Hence the economic growth until 1990 was relatively slow across the region.

India has been a key player in terms of economic growth contribution in the region. As such this region is Indo-centric because of the demography and its influence on development. The premise of HWB stems from concerted policies for welfare of people which is an important aspect of growth and development. India being the most populated country of the region has much greater influence on other countries of the region. Most of the economic activities in South Asia are influenced by the economic policies of India as it has a close economic relationship with all of its neighboring countries. Excepting Sri Lanka—which opened its economy in the latter part of 1970s—all other countries have implemented economic and trade liberalization reforms to respond to the changing international economic framework and fluctuating market conditions in latter part of 1980s and mid-1990s, after witnessing slow growth.

Facilitating economic liberalization included removing quantitative restrictions, moving to tariff system, lowering average nominal tariffs, narrowing the gap between nominal and effective tariffs, real devaluation of currency, unification of multiple exchange rates, removal of export taxes, and other restrictions and implementation of export subsidies. Earlier the economic policies were such that had lot of barriers on imports and exports. Liberalization of economic policies led to free trade among different countries resulting in creation of huge opportunities of growth of industry and services sector. Between 1995 and 1999, the average simple tariff rate in South Asia was the highest (around 25%) among all regions in the world (Bandara, 2009, p. 3). Apart from these indicative steps, several other initiatives were undertaken at national level.

Except Bhutan, all other South Asian countries are members of the World Trade Organization (WTO) and follow its terms, however, each nation individually designs its own trade policies to boost trade as per their requirements. Bhutan has expressed several reservations about joining the WTO. In 2017, a newspaper report[1] originating in Bhutan mentioned that Bhutan would not join WTO in the near future. There is a clear apprehension among Bhutan's government officials and ministers that the WTO is anti-GNH and if Bhutan becomes its member it would distract their focus from GNH. In the same newspaper report, the prime minister of Bhutan asked: "The question also is that do we really have the resources and the expertise to benefit from WTO?" Bhutan has a free trade agreement with both India and Bangladesh, which amounts to around 80% of its foreign trade. In the economics of Bhutan, hydro power has played a key role and contributed significantly to its GDP. In 2007, the contribution of electricity earnings to GDP was 23.4% (Kinga, 2009, p. 263). For the first time, electricity's contribution exceeded the contributions of the agriculture, livestock, and forestry sectors.

Afghanistan attempted to reduce their trade tariff and hence had the lowest tariff among all the countries in the region. Afghanistan developed close ties with European Union countries and thus benefited by the tariff preferences offered by those more developed countries. Bangladesh has also been able to reduce tariff rates and receive foreign direct investment (FDI) for its industrial growth initiatives. Sri Lanka opened its economy much before other countries of the region—in the late 1970s. This opening of the economy led to free trade policies with other countries and much of the import-export restrictions were lifted. Sri Lanka's GDP reflects the beneficial results from this decision and is thus more economically developed than other member countries of WTO from South Asia.

India's trade liberalization policy has helped ease FDI rules and over the last two decades it has largely been able to smoothen the process. The Maldives differs from its peers. Though small, this nation has been able to eliminate most of the trade barriers making it the most integrated economy of the region. Nepal and Pakistan both have also liberalized their economies and reduced tariff rates and quantitative restrictions. Their economies are also integrated, Pakistan has better economically developed as compared to Nepal, which has suffered from more political instabilities and inconsistent policies.

Relatively, South Asian economies have overall been less integrated with the other parts of the world. This was a blessing in disguise as the 2008 global financial crisis did not affect South Asia as strongly as other world regions. It does not mean that the efforts to become integrated with other parts of the world have not been made intentionally. The Indian economy has evolved significantly from 2008, and currently the high integration levels allow extensive economic exploration and is helping economy growth. FDI flows remained positive over last 27 years in India. In the preceding four years, India has succeeded in getting an FDI of USD $63 billion, the highest levels so far achieved.[2] The average time to clear exports through customs has been reduced from 15.1 days in 2006 to 5.8 days in 2014 by India, whereas the

---

[1] See news item captioned *Govt Says No To WTO For Now* available from https://thebhutanese.bt/govt-says-no-to-wto-for-now/ retrieved on 28.06.2018.

[2] This information is obtained from the website of Press Information Bureau, Govt of India which is available at http://pibarchive.nic.in/ndagov/Initiatives.aspx.

world average is 7.4 days, and the average in the South Asian region is 8.7 days.[3] This exemplifies the concern that the Indian government has for encouraging exports resulting in improved GDP.

Government's concern over improving trade is reflected through the improving data on trade, which examines the sum of exports and imports of goods and services (percent of GDP). Between 1990 and 2016, trade in South Asia has been prioritized by the regions governments, which has resulted in increasing trade by around 2 times. This has been even faster in case of India where increase in trade is by 2.5 times[4] leading to an indirect increase in GDP. Afghanistan registered more than 20,000 new businesses (limited liability companies or LLCs) in 2012 alone, which is second highest in South Asia. India had registered more than 100 thousand LLCs. The boom in new business reflects the encouragement governments were providing to entrepreneurs to start their own enterprises. This trend is reflected in the whole of South Asia. However, small countries like the Maldives and Bhutan had meagre growth in this regard.

To promote trade and industry in the region, the South Asia Preferential Trade Agreement (SAPTA) was signed in 1993, which in 2004 became South Asia Free Trade Agreement (SAFTA). All the countries of the region are members of SAFTA. These countries have both, bilateral preferential trade agreements with other South Asian countries as well as bilateral agreements and group agreements with countries outside of the South Asian region. India plays a major role negotiating and managing these agreements which is a part of its international economic diplomacy (Pursell, 2011, p. 221). "India is not only the dominant country of the region but also the most diversified economy in terms of trading partners and range of commodities traded" (Bhattarai, 2011, p. 262). These agreements have immensely helped all countries of the region boost their trade with neighboring nations as well as with more geographically disparate countries which has positively affected South Asian GDP growth. The GDP growth in the whole region has been impressive in last 27 years, which is the result of growth driven economic policies.

Demonetization and implementation of Goods and Services Tax (GST) by the government in India has been claimed (by the government) to have resulted in the positive economic growth of the country, though it also resulted in an uproar by the masses (especially demonetization) when it was introduced. These policies brought the informal sector on board by recording the transactions and broadening tax net. The policies have been able to push the use of technology as a facilitator for all kinds of transactions. Largely, demonetization has been able to reveal money scams and curb corruption to a great extent. One of the members of the Reserve Bank of India (the central bank of India), S. Gurumurthy, while appreciating policy said that:

---

[3] See World Bank, Enterprise Surveys (http://www.enterprisesurveys.org/) retrieved on November 14, 2018.

[4] See World Bank national accounts data, and OECD National Accounts data files from World Development Indicators retrieved on July 22, 2018.

In just 18 months prior to demonetization, 500 rupee, 1000 rupee (notes) rose to 4800 billion (4.8 lakh crore[5]) that is what funded the real estate and gold prices and we would have gone the same way, (as what happened in) 2008 in the US due to sub-prime lending… but for demonetization, the Indian economy would have collapsed. It was a corrective measure.[6]

The introduction of GST has been pending for the past several years, however in 2016 the government reexamined this initiative by taking all political parties into confidence and eventually introduced the One Nation, One Tax—One Nation, One Market policy, leading to the implementation of GST on July 1, 2017. All indirect taxes were brought under GST through four brackets of 5, 12, 18, and 28%. This policy has controlled inflation by reducing the cascading effect of taxes, reducing illegal transactions, and benefitting the consumer—besides reducing the multiplicity of taxes and simplifying procedures. This move is one of the biggest tax reforms ever implemented in India. According to rough estimates, the implementation of GST has helped GDP grow by around 2%.

Fiscal policies are an important part of economic planning for any country. More so for developing countries as they lack the same resources as more developed nations. Tax revenue in such countries is a major source of economic income to finance welfare measures. For all South Asian countries, the pressure for spending by different governments on fulfilling collective social wants (public expenditure) has been enormous as there are many areas where substantial expenditure is required. In high-income countries, the public expenditure to GDP ratio is almost twice as high as it is in South Asian countries. Even low- to middle-income countries had a higher public expenditure to GDP ratio than South Asian countries. Between 1995 and 2007, the public expenditure to GDP ratio rose in India but actually fell in Pakistan and Sri Lanka, partly because of the squeeze in revenue in these two countries (Jha, 2011, p. 172). The trend of the last 10 years shows a rise in public expenditure in all parts of the South Asia region.

In 2005, the Indian Parliament passed a historic law which guaranteed employment to the rural population (Box 3.1) entitled "National Rural Employment Guarantee Act, 2005." This improved the living conditions of rural populations by empowering them to seek employment when they would otherwise be idle. It has also resulted in an inflow of funds contributing to increasing consumption and demand. Considered to be a landmark scheme guaranteeing every rural household 100 days of work a year at a reasonable wage (Zepeda, McDonald, Panda, Kumar, & Sapkota, 2013), it indirectly also plays a role in correcting labor rates in the wage market.

---

[5]INR 1000 is equivalent to around USD 14.5.

[6]See *The Economic Times Daily*, Nov 15, 2018 retrieved from https://economictimes.indiatimes. com/news/politics-and-nation/economy-would-have-collapsed-but-for-demonetisation-s-gurumurthy/articleshow/66641864.cms.

Box 3.1

Brief about Mahatma Gandhi National Rural Employment Guarantee Act

Aiming to enhance the employment security for rural populations in India, "National Rural Employment Guarantee Act, 2005" was enforced in 2005 and was later renamed as "Mahatma Gandhi National Rural Employment Guarantee Act" (MGNREGA). This law works as a social security measure aimed towards providing at least 100 days of wage employment in a year to households who volunteer to work under the program. Other aims of MGNREGA include the creation of durable assets for the country in the form of roads, ponds, wells, etc.

It was first proposed by the then Prime Minister of India, Narasimha Rao in 1991, but would not see the light of the day until 2005. MGNREGA is regarded as "the largest and most ambitious social security and public works program in the world."[7] World Bank called it a 'stellar example of rural development'[8] in its report in 2014. MGNREGA works to improve the bargaining power of laborers who are often exposed to exploitative working conditions. Under the act, employment is provided within 5 kms of an applicant's residence and minimum wage is guaranteed. It also entitles a worker to an unemployment allowance for those who are not provided employment within 15 days of applying.[9]

MGNREGA also works to empower women, protect the environment, and foster social security and equity across India. The act aims to improve the purchasing power of rural people by focusing on the economic and social empowerment of women, by hiring women for roughly one-third of the workforce. Various activities under MGNREGA relate to agricultural and allied activities, watershed, irrigation and flood management works, agricultural and livestock related works, fisheries, works in coastal areas, and the rural drinking water and sanitation works. Implemented by the Gram Panchayats, minimum wages under MGNREGA vary from state to state. This is one of the world's largest employment programs in terms of its scale and architecture. It promotes integration between resource management and the generation

---

[7] An anthology of research studies on MGNREGA by the ministry of rural development, government of India for the period between 2006 and 2012 mentions this statement in its foreword. Available at https://web.archive.org/web/20130921125532/ http://nrega.nic.in/netnrega/writereaddata/Circulars/MGNREGA_SAMEEKSHA.pdf.

[8] As reported in the Indian daily the Economic Times: http://articles.economictimes.indiatimes.com/2013-10-10/news/42902947_1_world-bank-world-development-report-safety-net.

[9] See http://www.mgnrega.co.in/features-of-mnrega.htm.

of livelihood, and has revolutionized rural areas by improving the purchasing power of the rural population.

This program emphasizes the role of state as a provider of livelihoods within the reach of participants themselves. Under catastrophic circumstances such as flood, drought, or any other calamity, the provision of minimum number of days gets extended to provide more work. The program also features a social audit aspect in which parties involved under the act are put under scrutiny and inspection on a continuous basis is conducted. Even disabled individuals are made aware of the MGNREGA under the act. The workers are reached on the online web-based worksite and are instructed about the type of work that would be suitable for them such as arranging drinking water for workers, taking care of children, plantation, earth backfilling, digging of canals/irrigation, etc.

In the 2017–2018 fiscal year, INR 64,179 crore (approx. USD 14 billion) has been spent on this program, the highest in all the years since the act was adopted. More than 60% of the work performed was related to individual asset creation for sustainable livelihoods, which has played a key role in improving the well-being of the rural population. In order to directly reach to the beneficiaries, more than 96% of the total expenditure was directly transferred to the bank account of the beneficiaries.[10] This act has transformed the lives of villagers across India and has improved their general well-being through female empowerment, increased purchasing power, asset creation, reduction in labor migration, and building trust in the government.

Food-for-work programs in Bangladesh have helped the country alleviate poverty extensively since 1975, particularly for rural workers during the slack seasons. Each year they have provided 100 million workdays for over 4 million people (Muqtada, 1987). Bangladesh Rural Advancement Committee (BRAC) is one of the world's largest NGOs which has played a pivotal role in the uplift of marginalized populations. A brief profile of BRAC is provided in Box 3.2.

Box 3.2
Brief about Bangladesh Rural Advancement Committee (BRAC)
BRAC is an international non-government organization (NGO) started in Bangladesh for the purpose of development activities. It was established in 1972 by Sir Fazle Hasan Abed after Bangladesh gained its independence. As the largest NGO in the world, it employs over 100 thousand employees, 70% of which are women. It is present in all 64 districts of Bangladesh; it has its operations based in 12 countries across Asia, Africa, and America. Started as a small-scale relief and rehabilitation project for helping war refugees after

---

[10]See http://nrega.nic.in/netnrega/circular_new.aspx.

the Bangladesh Liberation War of 1971,[11] BRAC now reaches more than 126 million people around the world. With a vision of creating a world free from all forms of exploitation and discrimination where everyone has the opportunity to realize their potential,[12] it has established itself as a pioneer in recognizing and tackling different realities of poverty.

In the initial years of its operation, BRAC focused on community development through programs focusing on health, family planning, vocational training for women, agriculture, rural crafts, etc. Towards the latter part of 1970s it started taking a more focused approach by creating Village Organizations (VO) to assist the landless and marginalized farmers, artisans, and vulnerable women. Microfinance was one of the earliest programs of BRAC which focused on providing collateral-free loans to the landless and rural people of Bangladesh in order to improve their standard of living. BRAC has created a substantial impact by enabling access to financial services to over 5 million families. Today, it has 5.6 million active borrowers covering all districts in Bangladesh, and 87% of its clients are women.[13] It is the first organization in Bangladesh, and largest in the world, to be recognized with a Smart Certification for upholding universal standards for client protection as determined by the Smart Campaign.[14] Its education programs focus on primary education for the rural and deprived children as well as dropouts which resulted in improvements in female enrolment in primary schools and a reduction in the gap between male and female attendance in schools.[15]

With the motto of 'investing in the next generation', BRAC works on providing a low cost, scalable schooling model making it the largest secular private education provider in the world. With their efforts, 1.8 million students are enrolled in schools and 1.4 million youth are engaged in reading, socializing, and learning in Bangladesh. BRAC's contribution in the field of health care has also been remarkable. Their community-based health care approach employs numerous community workers to ensure that poor people, have access to high-quality and affordable health services. It has built a strong network which connects communities to public and private health services and provides low-cost health packages to meet their basic needs. BRAC also follows a proactive approach for climate changes and emergencies. It conducts

---

[11] See https://www.hbs.edu/creating-emerging-markets/interviews/Pages/profile.aspx?profile=fhabed.

[12] See http://www.brac.net/our-approach.

[13] See http://www.brac.net/program/wp-content/uploads/2018/08/BRAC-Microfinance-Factsheet-29.08.2018.pdf.

[14] See Footnote 13.

[15] See http://rih.stanford.edu/rosenfield/resources/Primary%20Education%20in%20Bangladesh.pdf.

predictive researches, transfers information, educates communities, and generally increases the coping abilities in case of natural disasters.[16] Its programs holistically respond to unforeseen disasters and promote better disaster management, adaption strategies, and knowledge generation.

BRAC has also worked for decades to eliminate gender injustice. Its gender equality and diversity programs work on improving gender relations, empowering women, eliminating violence against women, and promoting gender justice in Bangladesh and world.[17] Bangladesh Girl Summit in 2014 hosted by BRAC focused on the menace of child marriage and provoked national and international support on this subject. Strengthening the capacity of civil society, BRAC formed the Sexual Harassment Elimination (SHE) policy in 2004 that enforced "Mon Khule Kotha Bola" or "to listen to the voice of the staff" forum in order to enable a friendly and communicative environment within the organization and continued to review and update their policies and programs for gender justice and protection of women's rights.

It is important to note that the background of its founder has provided BRAC with a foundation to establish various social enterprises which are self-sustaining business enterprises, creating a social impact and reinvesting the surplus to increase that impact. Some of its ventures include "Aarong" which is Bangladesh's largest retail chain that harnesses the skill of nearly 65,000 artisans.[18] Similarly, 'BRAC chicken' is one of the largest automated poultry processing plants in Bangladesh and supplies high quality chicken and frozen food products to the public.[19] BRAC also invests in various socially responsible companies that assist them in their mission to empower people and communities in situations of poverty, illiteracy, disease, and social injustice and help work toward self-sustainability. Recently, BRAC has signed a MoU with the National Human Rights Commission (NHRC) to increase the facilities for the disabled in the metro rail system.[20]

In 2001, BRAC established the BRAC University whose goal was to foster national development through excellence in higher education that is also responsive to the needs of society.[21] It is the top ranked private university in Bangladesh, actively concentrating on developing the creation of

---

[16]See http://www.brac.net/dmcc.

[17]See http://www.brac.net/gender.

[18]See http://www.brac.net/brac-enterprises/item/878-aarong.

[19]See https://www.brac.net/brac-enterprises/item/880-brac-chicken.

[20]Retrieved from http://www.brac.net/latest-news/item/1180-brac-and-nhrc-sign-mou-to-increase-facility-for-persons-with-disabilities-in-metro-rail.

[21]See https://www.bracu.ac.bd/ for details.

knowledge and learning attitude. BRAC has been ranked as the number one NGO in the world by NGO advisors both in 2016 and 2017.[22] Out of more than 500 organizations worldwide, NGO Advisor placed BRAC first in its international category, based on its impact, innovation, and sustainability.

BRAC has been the recipient of numerous awards such as the AGFUND International Prize for Pioneering Human Development Projects and OFID Annual Award for Development in 2018.[23] It continues to work towards human well-being by empowering people and communities suffering from poverty, illiteracy, disease, and social injustice while upholding its core values of integrity, innovation, inclusiveness, and effectiveness. The future citizens of the world and of Bangladesh in particular will greatly benefit from the contributions of BRAC.

The limited availability of money has been one of the major barriers to converting an idea into reality. In the absence of education and social security, it further becomes more challenging to qualify for loans from the traditional banks or other lending institutions. In this given environment, Muhammad Yunus (Box 3.3), a professor in Bangladesh took initiative and formed Grameen Bank which, through microfinancing, revolutionized the small finance loan eco-system. Grameen Bank has positively affected the general well-being of people in Bangladesh and has influenced many other countries to follow suit. The contribution of Yunus is extraordinary in the realm of poverty alleviation and improving the financial well-being of a historically disadvantaged section of the population in Bangladesh as well as in other countries where micro financing[24] is practiced. Bangladesh's microfinance institutions (MFI) have recorded impressive growth in the last two and a half decades and have successfully contributed to societal inclusivity. "By 2016, it had more than 750 registered MFIs with a network of over 17,000 branches…by 2013, some 32 million MFI members had received more than USD 7.2 billion in annual disbursements, with an outstanding balance of USD 4.5 billion equivalent to 3% of GDP" (Khandker, Khalily, & Samad, 2016, p. 237). Bangladesh has played a key role in spreading the success story of microcredit for all developing nations where small credit is needed and used.

---

[22]Read about this news http://www.brac.net/component/k2/item/978-brac-ranked-number-one-ngo-in-the-world.

[23]Read about all the awards and recognitions http://www.brac.net/recognition?view=page.

[24]Micro financing is a banking service which was initially meant for people belonging to poor and/or marginalised section of society who did not have access to formal banking system. However now Micro Financing Institutions operate as non-banking financial corporations, providing loan to other people as well.

Box 3.3

Brief Profile of Muhammad Yunus

Muhammad Yunus, pioneer in microfinance, is the founder of Grameen Bank in Bangladesh and is credited with the idea of micro credit. He understood the significant difference a small loan could make in the lives of poor people who were often not served by the traditional banks due to the high risk of default. In 1982, Grameen bank started its operations as a full-fledged bank for poor Bangladeshis.[25] Yunus' persistent efforts for ensuring human well-being not only helped millions in Bangladesh but also millions across the world. The ability to obtain a loan for the poverty stricken who had no financial security was a distant dream until the establishment of Grameen Bank which was instrumental in ensuring social and economic development for Bangladesh. Yunus transformed his vision into reality and proved that poorest of poor can work together for their own upliftment.

In 2006, he became Bangladesh's first Nobel Prize winner. The success story of Grameen Bank led to similar efforts in more than 100 developing countries around the world and the Grameen Social Business Model (GSBM) has been transformed from a theory to practice. Yunus firmly believed that credit is a fundamental human right and acts as a catalyst for escaping poverty, promoting self-sufficiency, and boosting economic development. He received numerous awards for his ideas and endeavors like the Mohamed Shabdeen Award for Science (1993) in Sri Lanka, the Humanitarian Award (1993) by CARE, USA, the World Food Prize (1994) by World Food Prize Foundation, USA, Seoul Peace Prize (2006), and Bangladesh's highest civilian award—the King Hussein Humanitarian Leadership Award (2000).[26] He was also awarded the United States Presidential Medal of Freedom in 2009 and the Congressional Gold Medal in 2010[27] and KISS Humanitarian Award in 2018.[28]

He is a member of the International Advisory Group for the Fourth World Conference on Women and on the board of the United Nations Foundation.[29] He also served on the Global Commission of Women's Health, the Advisory Council for Sustainable Economic Development, and the UN Expert Group on Women and Finance.[30] In 2008, Texas declared January 14th as

---

[25] See http://grameenresearch.org/history-of-grameen-bank/ for details.

[26] See https://www.nobelprize.org/prizes/peace/2006/yunus/biographical/.

[27] See　　　　　　https://www.speaker.gov/press-release/house-senate-leaders-announce-gold-medal-ceremony-professor-muhammad-yunus.

[28] See　　https://www.business-standard.com/article/pti-stories/prof-muhammad-yunus-conferred-kiss-humanitarian-award-2018-118051100725_1.html.

[29] See　　https://unfoundation.org/media/nobel-laureate-muhammad-yunus-joins-mhealth-alliance-board/.

[30] See https://www.nobelprize.org/prizes/peace/2006/yunus/biographical/.

'Muhammad Yunus Day' to honor his contribution in uplifting poverty through his micro-finance initiative.[31] He was named among the World's 50 Most Influential Figures in 2010[32] and as one of the greatest entrepreneurs of the current era by Fortune Magazine in 2012.[33]

He has received 50 honorary doctorate degrees from universities of various countries such as the UK, US, Canada, Australia, India, Japan, etc.[34] He was the subject of two documentaries titled To *Catch a dollar* in 2010 and *Bonsai people—The vision of Muhammad Yunus* in 2011.[35] He authored several books including *Building social business: The new kind of capitalism that serves humanity's most pressing needs* in 2010 and *A world of three zeroes: The new economics of zero poverty, zero unemployment, and zero net carbon emissions* in 2017.[36]

The Yunus Centre based in Dhaka—chaired by Prof. Yunus—functions as a think tank for social business issues and works extensively towards eradicating poverty and ensuring sustainability and human well-being.[37] His unparalleled vision for transforming small savings and investments into big venture financing has shown a path of economic empowerment to poor people and has contributed towards improving the living conditions of innumerous people around the globe. The South Asian region has benefitted by the myriad efforts of Muhammad Yunus and his strong commitment towards eradicating poverty through small banking solutions, which will keep guiding the efforts of many in the region as well as globally.

Nepal's Emergency Employment Programme, targeted towards marginalized communities, covered roughly 5% of the population to meet the post-conflict need for employment and a peace dividend (Langer, Stewart, & Venugopal, 2012). These initiatives have helped marginalized communities residing in remote and rural areas to improve their well-being to a larger extent.

In the next part of this chapter, GDP spent on education and health and other qualitative policy initiatives shall be discussed to relate with the outcomes that have been discussed in Chap. 2.

---

[31]See   http://www.muhammadyunus.org/index.php/media/in-the-media/191-january-14-as-muhammad-yunus-day.

[32]See https://www.newstatesman.com/global-issues/2010/09/loan-star-yunus-bangladesh.

[33]See https://web.archive.org/web/20120324163515/ http://money.cnn.com/galleries/2012/news/companies/1203/gallery.greatest-entrepreneurs.fortune/13.html.

[34]See http://muhammadyunus.org/index.php/professor-yunus/awards?limitstart=0.

[35]See   https://www.nytimes.com/2012/02/10/movies/bonsai-people-a-documentary-about-muhammad-yunus.html.

[36]See https://www.thriftbooks.com/a/muhammad-yunus/198251/.

[37]See https://www.theguardian.com/sustainable-business/2017/mar/29/we-are-all-entrepreneurs-muhammad-yunus-on-changing-the-world-one-microloan-at-a-time.

3.3   Policies for Education Well-Being

In April 2000, the World Education Forum began a program called Education For All (EFA), whose purpose was to provide primary education to all children in the world by 2015. The United Nations Educational, Scientific and Cultural Organization (UNESCO) led this global movement and created awareness among all nations about the initiative. It was a major challenge for many global regions, particularly for African countries as well as for South Asian nations. The goals of EFA strengthened the Millennium Development Goals (MDGs), which were to also achieve universal primary education and gender equality in education by 2015. While reviewing the progress in 2015, it was found that the South Asia region was far behind the other regions on attaining EFA status. The Sustainable Development Goals (SDGs) replaced MDGs in 2015 and stated for quality education. The attainment of EFA status was reiterated by the UN. The South Asian countries were to provide more time and effort in order to attain EFA status.

All the governments in the South Asian region have been working to strengthen their educational systems. The first important step towards this was to invest in education. The financial allocations made by the countries of the region are discussed hereunder, followed by a focused narrative on the different policies enhancing the education sector as a whole. Low achievement and slow progress in education in this region is attributable to the fact that South Asian countries have spent less on education than other countries at a similar level of development (Martin, Béteille, Li, Mitra, & Newman, 2015, p. 20). General government expenditure on education (current, capital, and transfers) is expressed as a percentage of GDP. In 2010, the GDP spent on education in South Asia was only 2.5%, whereas the global average was 4.5% (Table 3.1). As per latest available data of 2016, The Maldives had the highest

Table 3.1   Government expenditure (GDP share in percentage)

	1991	1996	2001	2006	2011	2016
Afghanistan	NA	NA	NA	NA	3.44	3.24[g]
Bangladesh	1.43	1.95[a]	2.17	2.13	2.13	2.50
Bhutan	NA	NA	5.72	7.08[e]	4.65	7.39[g]
India		3.41[a]	4.38[b]	3.19	3.84	3.84[h]
The Maldives	NA	NA	5.79[c]	4.65	3.51	4.25
Nepal	NA	NA	3.71	3.61	3.84	3.70[g]
Pakistan	2.57	2.81	1.84[b]	2.63	2.22	2.49
Sri Lanka	2.92	3.34	3.05[d]	2.06[f]	1.81	3.49
South Asia	2.57	3.02	2.55[b]	2.91	2.83	2.50
World	NA	NA	4.09	4.19	4.49	4.89[i]

a: 1997; b: 2000; c: 2002; d: 1998; e: 2005; f: 2009; g: 2015; h: 2013; i: 2014
Source Compiled from world development indicators data retrieved on 24.11.18 from http://databank.worldbank.org/data/source/world-development-indicators

allocation in the region at 4.25% followed by Sri Lanka (3.49%).[38] This level of expenditure is very well reflected as these two countries are the most literate countries, and they have been able to sustain this relatively high rate of literacy over the last five decades. India spent 3.84% of GDP on education in 2013 (the last available data), compared to Pakistan who spent the lowest at 2.76% in 2017. It is important to observe that in some countries GDP spent on education has declined over the past several years. This is the case for India which spent 4.48% in 1999 and reduced that to 3.31% in 2009. Similarly, Nepal also reduced its expenditure on education from 5.79% in 2002 to 4.25% in 2016. These are challenging times for nations aspiring to improve well-being as they need to organize their priorities strategically and prioritize expenditure on education.

Total government expenditure on education as a percentage of GDP reflects the priority of the government. Governmental expenditure on education includes current, capital, and transfers as well as fund transfers from international sources to local, regional, or/and central governments. Globally on an average, countries spend around 5% of their GDP on education. Surprisingly this spend is too low in this region, almost at around half of the world rate (Fig. 3.1) whereas ideally it should be spending more as it is a relatively underdeveloped region. The trend as depicted in Fig. 3.1 provides

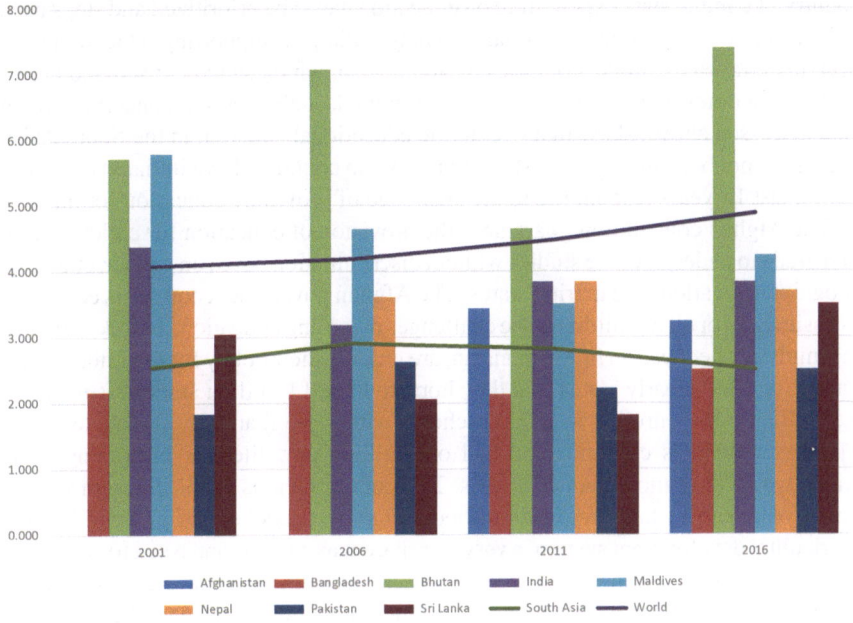

Fig. 3.1 Expenditure on education as part of GDP

---

[38] As depicted in Table 3.1, data for 2016 is available for Bangladesh, the Maldives, Pakistan, and Sri Lanka. However, for Afghanistan, Bhutan and Nepal it is of 2015 and that of India is of 2013. Hence for comparison here, only 2016 data is compared. It is observed that in 2015, Bhutan had largest allocation at 7.39% of GDP for education.

an evidence that the gap between expenditure on education (out of GDP) by the world and by the South Asian countries is widening. The expenditure on education by South Asian governments is on a decreasing trend since last more than a decade whereas the world has been increasing its proportion of expenditure on education.

Mean and expected years of schooling data have been explained in the last chapter at length. Broadly, the governments of the South Asia region have been putting efforts towards improving expected years and mean years of schooling. There have been improvements on these indicators in last two decades time. There have been changes in the policy of some countries of the region on the duration of compulsory education. Afghanistan has increased compulsory education years from six (1998) to nine in 2017 which is helping improve literacy levels. Bangladesh has the fewest number of compulsory education years at five, which has remained constant for several years. India has made it to eight mandatory years by enacting the RTE Act. Pakistan mandates 12 years of compulsory education whereas Sri Lanka specifies nine years. The world average and the average of South Asia is the same at nine years. Compulsory educational years is an important input in examining education policy which is reflected by improving educational levels. It is interesting to note that of the total teachers in secondary education in the world, around 14% are in India. India has the third largest higher education system in the world. For the size of the country like India, state expenditure on education has to be prioritized and steps need to be taken in order to improve quality. Many initiatives supporting education have been undertaken by all the countries of South Asia, which shall be discussed here.

The outcomes in education as discussed in the last chapter and concerning input data discussed above, show that overall the educational situation in the South Asian region has not been impressive. Many South Asian countries have initiated programs during last 15 years responding to the challenge of providing education for all.

The Afghan constitution guarantees the provision of education for children from first grade to undergraduate studies without discrimination based on gender, ethnicity, geographic location, and marital status. The Afghan government considers education as basic right for all its children. The challenges regarding education, as understood by the ministry of education in Afghanistan, are guiding their policy for the future. Their vision for 2020 clearly states that they hope to have 14 million students (including 6.5 million girls) enrolled in 22,000 schools with more than 50% female teachers. The government is committed to add one million new literates in coming years which would have more than 60% girls. This commitment is visible through various initiatives taken in last few years to boost literacy, especially of girl child. Their curriculum development system is very transparent as citizens are asked to contribute to the draft which is put on the web for public opinion. They have also stated that technical and vocational education will be integrated into both general and Islamic schools.[39]

---

[39]The information regarding developments in Afghanistan has been retrieved from official website of the Ministry of Education, Government of Afghanistan (http://moe.gov.af/en/page/2020).

Bangladesh legislated the right to education through the Compulsory Primary Education Act in 1990, which resulted in achieving a gross enrolment rate in primary schools of 100%. Bangladesh designed programs for inclusive education for students with special needs (Malak, 2013). To improve teacher training, equity, quality, and access, it initiated programs such as Teaching Quality Improvement in Secondary Education Project in 2005, Secondary Education Quality and Access Enhancement Project in 2008, and Higher Secondary Female Stipend Project in 2009. The National Education Policy was introduced in 2010 to reform education delivery mechanisms and the Third Primary Education Development Program was launched in 2011. The education policy encompassed broader goals including improvement in the intellectual and practical qualities of the learners by focusing on moral, human, cultural, scientific, and social values. Their commitment to create a society free from the curse of illiteracy is quite visible through this policy. Interestingly, the policy document mentions the tolerance of corporate life (lavish life style) and love for honest living, friendliness, and perseverance which is in line with the larger goal of human life, namely happiness and peace. The state's concern for encouraging thinking, imagination, creativity, practicability, and productivity for economic and social development and developing a scientific mindset is also included in their educational goals. Avoidance of rote learning, acquiring skills for self-employment, and use of ICT (Information and Computer Technology) in education is also highlighted in the policy.

The Bangladesh government published a National Skill Development Policy in 2011[40] to focus on technical and vocational education and training, aiming to strengthen the Bangladesh Technical Education Board which regulates and monitors technical education. They were able to achieve 97% net enrolment rate for primary education which is an important achievement in the light of SDGs and EFA goals.

Bhutan as a young democratic nation has been able to improve its education indicators. The Bhutan Education Development Project was initiated in 2003 to boost enrolment of children up to the tenth grade. All of the Five-Year Plans (FYPs) that have been introduced thus far, mention of education as a key priority. This priority is reflected through their GDP share expenditure on education as discussed before. The Bhutan 2020 Document as prepared by the Planning Commission (1999) clearly states that "Education must prepare young people for the world of work and instill an acceptance on the dignity of labor" (p. 19). The 32nd Education Policy Guidelines and Instructions 2018[41] under the ministry of education, provide details of future plans for education. The ministry introduced Early Childhood Care and Development (ECCD) program to foster creative, intellectual and social development of children apart from enhancing their school readiness and preparedness for effective lifelong learning. The ministry has made concerted efforts to improve access to quality and inclusive

---

[40] This information is gathered through EFA report prepared by Bangladesh government and submitted to UNESCO. The report is available at http://unesdoc.unesco.org/images/0023/002305/230507e.pdf.

[41] See PPD (2018), the details retrieved on November 18, 2018 from http://www.education.gov.bt/downloads/epgi.pdf.

ECCD. From five centers in 2006, Bhutan now has 307 ECCD centers, including those run by NGOs, private bodies, and corporations. In the 12th FYP (2018–2023), the ministry plans to enroll at least 50% of children aged 3–5 years in ECCD centers. It has shown true commitment to improving inclusive education through specialized centers (Special Education Needs—SEN program) for differently-abled persons. At present, it has 16 schools with SEN programs across the country providing benefits to more than 600 children enrolled in them. Through implementation of the 12th FYP, it hopes to improve access for all children with special needs by identifying at least one school with SEN program in every *Dzongkhags* (district) and *Thromdes* (second-level administrative division after district). It has been made mandatory for all private schools to be headed by competent Bhutanese nationals only. The weight of school bags is standardized and the fitness and hygiene levels for all cooks working in schools is made mandatory. The state's commitment to health and well-being of students and other citizens are reflected through its policies and actions.

The government of India launched three important flagship initiatives to boost the education sector as a whole. To achieve universal elementary enrolment and retention by 2010, *Sarva Shiksha Abhiyan*[42] (SSA) was conceived and implemented from 2002 onwards. This initiative was strongly supported by the World Bank. The primary focus of SSA has been to increase enrolment in primary schools. SSA also recruited and trained teachers, provided textbooks and teaching materials, and monitored learning outcomes. Its programs have annually benefited around 130 million children in government schools and another 17 million enrolled in government-aided private schools. Roughly 71 million girls, 27 million children from India's disadvantaged groups, 15 million tribal children, and 2.8 million children with special needs have gained access to education because of SSA. SSA outcomes have contributed to the governmental push to enact a national right to education law in order to guarantee free and compulsory basic education for all children (World Bank, 2013, p. 6).

In order to expand the number of secondary schools necessary to ensure universal enrolment for the ninth and tenth grades by 2018, *Rashtriya Madhyamik Shiksha Abhiyan*[43] was launched in 2009. In the same year, the Indian Parliament passed the Right to Education Act, which mandated free compulsory education for all children between the ages of 6 and 14. This act mandates a minimum school infrastructure such as a building, a library, toilets, and an appropriate pupil-to-teacher ratio. This act is one of the landmark decisions to improve the enrolment rate, and thus far it has been able to positively affect the enrolment rate.[44] In 2013, *Rashtriya Uchchatar Shiksha Abhiyan*[45] (RUSA) was launched to improve the overall quality of state institutions and provide funds to institutions of higher education run by state governments. It also focused on reforms in higher education administration and processes, and worked to create suitable environments to promote research and innovation. A total of 384 state

---

[42]Education For All Movement.

[43]National Secondary Education Movement.

[44]The national gross enrolment ratio (2012) prior to the launch of RUSA was 20.8 (male 22.1 and female 19.4) which has increased to 24.5 (male 25.4 and female 23.5) in 2015–2016.

[45]National Higher Education Movement.

public universities and more than 13,000 colleges across different states and union territories are covered under RUSA.[46] The funding is supposed to be norm-based and outcome-oriented. At present India has around 40,000 colleges spread across the country. More than half of this number has only been added in last 18 years.

The current Indian government which came to power in 2014, has undertaken many initiatives to improve education accessibility, quality, and gender equity during its tenure. In last four years, it has been able to offer scholarships to more than seven hundred thousand students enrolled in different schools and colleges. The amount of scholarships given to students in higher education has reached INR 1273 crore (approx. USD 180 million).[47] In order to develop leadership qualities among youth a new program was launched under five different categories as, 1. Neighborhood Youth Parliament, 2. Youth for Development Program, 3. National Young Leaders Award, 4. National Youth Advisory Council, and 5. National Youth Development Fund. This initiative has attracted active participation of youth from all parts of the country. In 2016, drafting of the National Policy on Education was initiated. Currently a revised draft has been prepared by the government titled "Draft National Education Policy 2019". The government has invited comments and suggestions from all stakeholders by putting it in public domain.[48] It is expected that within 2019, new education policy shall be implemented. There have been many reforms in administering the university system and focusing on quality of higher education through emphasizing objectivity and performance measurement.

Nepal experience in improving educational standards is very interesting. Community schools were initially run by the communities themselves; however, the central government of Nepal took them over and initiated efforts to improve the system and its delivery. This initiative backfired, and in 2001 the Education Act was amended to return the management of schools back to the communities (Dundar, Beteille, Riboud, & Deolalikar, 2014, p. 358). Nepal initiated the Basic Primary Education Project, the Community School Support Program, the Secondary Education Support Program, and the Education for All Program to improve the enrolment rate and implement the universalization of education at different levels. In 2009, the School Sector Reform Program was launched to improve the quality of education for primary and middle school children. These initiatives helped the country to improve its educational parameters.

The School Sector Development Plan (2016/17–2022/23)[49] of the ministry of education, science, and technology focuses on improving equity, quality, efficiency, governance and management, and resilience through various initiatives it has taken to improve overall education accessibility and standards. Through these initiatives,

---

[46] Detailed guidelines of RUSA are available at http://rusa.nic.in/wp-content/uploads/2018/04/draft-guidelines.pdf.

[47] This information is obtained from the website of Press Information Bureau, Govt of India available at http://pibarchive.nic.in/ndagov/Initiatives.aspx.

[48] The draft is available for comments and suggestions at https://mhrd.gov.in/sites/upload_files/mhrd/files/Draft_NEP_2019_EN_Revised.pdf.

[49] The information is obtained from the website of Ministry of Education, Science and Technology, Government of Nepal [https://moe.gov.np/article/1008/educational-brochures-2017.html].

Nepal is optimistic in their ability to achieve a 94% gross enrolment ratio at primary level by 2023.

The education parameters of Pakistan are lower than most of the other countries in the region. In 1992, the National Education Policy worked to raise literacy rate to 70% and identified its focus areas as the use of Quranic literacy, involvement of universities, emphasis on rural and urban slum areas, use of electronic media, and evening shifts in primary schools. The 8th FYP stated that education is an indispensable ingredient of development and a fundamental right of every individual and as Ahsan (2003, pp. 266–267) mentions, it also stated that almost half of the girls and one-fifth of boys between five and nine years of age are not enrolled in primary school, and adult literacy rate is barely 35%. The government has been emphasizing the importance of education through different policies but its financial allocation has been meagre (Ahsan, 2003, p. 276). In 2017, again the National Education Policy[50] was announced by the ministry of federal education and professional training. The policy document also mentions that Pakistan has a history of developing detailed and well-designed education policies since 1947 but has fallen short of implementing them. Some of the key policy highlights are:

- Promotion of technical and vocational education.
- Introduction of skills training at adult literacy centers.
- Access to higher education from its current level of 1.4 million students to 5 million students in next 5 years.
- Capacity building for all personnel involved in education.
- Introduction of new disciplines in the areas of emerging science and technology.
- Increase in the access to distance education.
- Increase in enrolment in science, technology, and vocational disciplines.
- Encourage and facilitate quality private sector education.
- Promoting use of ICT.
- Allocating 4% of GDP for education and training from 2018 onwards.

In terms of female education in Pakistan, the contributions of Malala Yousufzai (Box 3.4) are memorable and inspiring. As a young girl she defied the Taliban[51] and continued her quest for education and by speaking for the right to education for women. She has been an educational ambassador by creating awareness among the masses (particularly girls), urging them to become educated and thus empowered. For her courage and commitment to the cause she was awarded a Nobel Peace Prize in 2014.

---

[50]This information has been taken from the National Education Policy 2017–2025 document available at: http://www.moent.gov.pk/userfiles1/file/National%20Educaiton%20Policy%202017.pdf.

[51]As per Oxford Dictionary it is defined as: "A fundamentalist Muslim movement whose militia took control of much of Afghanistan from early 1995, and in 1996 took Kabul and set up an Islamic state. The Taliban were overthrown by US-led forces and Afghan groups in 2001 following the events of September 11." Accessed from https://en.oxforddictionaries.com/definition/taliban.

Box 3.4

Brief Profile of Malala Yousufzai

Education helps improve living conditions and empowers poor people to become self-sufficient. It is believed that educating a woman leads to educating a family. Education is a significant differentiator, especially in regions affected by terrorist activities. The South Asian region in general, and Afghanistan and Pakistan in particular, have experienced the challenge of dealing with terrorism and the difficulty in eliminating sectarian groups that are engaged in terrorist activities. The Taliban is one such terrorist organization which has caused serious disturbances in the region. In these troubled regions and times, the story of Malala Yousufzai is very inspiring.

The youngest Nobel laureate is the courageous teenager from Pakistan who became a symbol of defiance against the Taliban. At a young age of 11, Malala took on Taliban subjugation by giving voice to her passion for education. In 2007, the Taliban invaded Swat valley in Northwest Pakistan and imposed strict laws such as shutting down or destroying girls' schools, banning women from pursuing any active role in the society, carrying out suicidal bombings, by enforcing harsh punishments and killing of those who defied their orders. The state of anarchy in the Swat region compelled natives to either leave it or continue to live in miserable conditions. However, the Pakistani teenager continued to raise her voice for the right to education and fellow well-being. She was awarded Pakistan's first National Youth Peace Prize in 2011.[52]

With her continued efforts to protect the education of girls in Pakistan, Malala was on the hit list of Taliban militants who shot her on her way back from school. The assassination attempt led to protests and the ratification of Pakistan's first Right to Education Bill in 2012.[53] Her fighting spirit helped her survive the attack and she was honored with the launch of UNESCO Malala Fund for Girls' Right to Education. The government of Pakistan committed USD 10-million for this fund. Vital Voices Global Partnership also established the "Malala" fund to support education for all girls around the world.[54] Among the many awards, Malala won the United Nations Human Rights Prize and was named one of the most influential people in 2013 by Times Magazine. She became the youngest person to receive the Liberty Medal, a medal awarded by the National Constitution Center in Philadelphia to public figures striving for people's freedom throughout the world.[55] Her continued daring efforts to

---

[52] See https://www.britannica.com/biography/Malala-Yousafzai.

[53] See https://www.brookings.edu/blog/up-front/2013/04/08/quiet-progress-for-education-in-pakistan/.

[54] See https://www.vitalvoices.org/people/malala-yousafzai/.

[55] See https://constitutioncenter.org/blog/malala-yousafzai-receives-liberty-medal-in-philadelphia/.

support the right to education and to stand against the atrocities of the Taliban brought these issues into the limelight and exposed the violence of the Taliban.

In 2014, Malala became the youngest recipient of Nobel Peace Prize.[56] Her belief that "the pen is mightier than the sword" is reflected in her persistent efforts to provide education for all. She strives for peace and human well-being and understands the importance education plays in achieving it. She authored two books titled *I am Malala: How one girl stood up for education and changed the world* in 2014 and *Malala's magic pencil* in 2017. These books became popular among young readers and inspire and encourage girls not to succumb to societal pressure and receive an education. A documentary titled *He named me Malala* made by Davis Guggenheimin 2015[57] won him BAFTA award for best documentary.

She was instrumental in opening a girls' school in Lebanon for the refugees in the Syrian war. Today, the Malala Fund has its presence across various developing countries supporting education. It aims to recruit female teachers and eliminate gender discrimination in order to increase the number of girls enrolled in schools in Afghanistan. In Brazil, it helps women speak out for their rights and ensure that schools are accessible to the most marginalized girls. Campaigning for free, safe, and quality education for every girl is their foremost objective in countries like Nigeria and India.[58] Currently, Malala is studying at Oxford University and working as an education activist for the millions of girls who are out of school. She believes that education is a powerful weapon and one child, one teacher, one pen, and one book can change the world.[59]

The Maldives boasts the best adult literacy rate in the region. It has almost reached to the level of complete literacy. The country has been expanding its education network at all levels including teacher education and introducing reforms in curricula. Double shift schools having morning and evening shifts, are not able to engage students effectively, which prompted a reform to have single shift schools currently. The country has also implemented a decentralization and privatization strategy in order to address their lack of resources. Vocational education has also been emphasized in the Maldives.

When it comes to social indicators, or HDI, in the South Asia region, Sri Lanka is an outlier as it has achieved excellent results in improving health and education. Education is free from primary to university level and the medium of instruction is in Sinhalese or Tamil (their mother tongue). The goals as identified by the Sri

---

[56] See https://www.nobelprize.org/prizes/peace/2014/press-release/.

[57] See https://www.oscars.org/news/15-documentary-features-advance-2015-oscarr-race.

[58] See https://www.malala.org/gulmakai-network.

[59] See https://theirworld.org/explainers/malala-yousafzais-speech-at-the-youth-takeover-of-the-united-nations.

Lankan national system of education[60] should be the model for an ideal citizen for any country. These goals determine broader education policy in Sri Lanka and are very important. They are:

- Developing a Sri Lankan citizen with love and dedication to motherland through fostering national cohesion, national integrity, and national unity.
- Respecting human dignity, recognizing pluralistic nature and cultural diversity in Sri Lanka, upholding tolerance and reconciliation.
- Recognizing and conserving the worthy elements of the nation's heritage while responding to the challenges of a changing world.
- Creating and supporting an environment imbued with the values of social justice and a democratic way of life.
- Promoting a life style based on respect for human values and sustainable development.
- Promoting the physical, mental, and emotional well-being of individuals.
- Cultivating the attributes of a well-integrated and balanced personality.
- Developing human resources for productive work that enhances the quality of life of the individual and the nation to contribute to economic development.
- Empowering individuals to adapt to and manage change, and to develop capacity to cope with rapid change, complexities and unforeseen situations.
- Fostering a liberated world view in keeping with modern knowledge to secure a respectable place in global community.

In 2013, the ministry of education issued a document entitled "Education First," which lists the primary strategies and action plan for educational policy and helps enable Sri Lanka to meet the above goals. Some of the key strategies are:

- Free education in all government and assisted schools; grants to children with special needs and those from marginalized families; free textbooks to all students from Grade 1 to 11; free school uniform materials to all children from Grade 1 to 13; bursaries to 15,000 children from needy families annually on the results of Grade 5 examination; subsidized public transport for all children travelling in public transport; and a mid-day meal for children in disadvantaged primary and small schools.
- Implementation of compulsory education regulations; advocacy campaigns on compulsory education; increase in non-formal education (NFE) centers for out-of-school children; expand and improve the quality of vocational training centers; establish adult and community learning centers; and, develop and strengthen monitoring and evaluation framework for NFE.
- Increase in grants to *pirivenas*[61] for subsidizing the construction of special spaces; increase in grants to *pirivenas* for purchase of equipment; strengthen the teaching

---

[60]This information is taken from the official website of National Education Council, available at: http://nec.gov.lk/wp-content/uploads/2017/12/Towards-a-New-Education-Act.pdf.

[61]Pirivenas are traditional educational institutes which offer training to Buddhist clergy and lay students who wish to pursue education in a Buddhist environment.

of classical oriental languages and foreign languages; equip all schools with drinking water and sanitary facilities; accredit all schools using the criteria of health promoting schools; and strengthen skills-based health education.

Education has been an important agenda item of the SAARC. Since its formation in 1983, the eight member nations have discussed education and developed cooperative projects through different committees and regional centers located within member countries.[62] The SAARC Human Resource Development Centre was opened in Pakistan for the benefit of all the member states to undertake research, provide training, and disseminate information on human resource development issues.

Although South Asia is still the most illiterate region in the world, literacy rates have risen in last three decades. However, learning outcomes and the average level of skill acquisition are still low in both absolute and relative terms. Mean student achievements in mathematics, reading, and language are low throughout the region, excepting Sri Lanka; a large number of children do not master basic primary-school skills even by Grade 5 (Dundar et al., 2014, p. 86).

The desire of South Asian governments to improve access to education as well as the quality of education has been the basis for all educational policies. But these nations, excepting Bhutan, have not appropriated sufficient expenditure on education as a whole to achieve these goals. The trend of educational expense from the whole South Asian region (Fig. 3.1) is going down whereas the world share of GDP provisions for education has been consistently rising.

3.4   Policies for Health Well-Being

The mission to achieve "HealthFor All" was initiated by the World Health Organization (WHO) in 1977[63] intending to provide good primary health facilities to all to improve the personal state of well-being. The WHO identified key areas such as the elimination of malnutrition, medical ignorance, contaminated drinking water, unhygienic housing, and the scarcity of doctors, hospital beds, and vaccines. The WHO required that health spending be a priority in government expenditure and all stakeholders participate in recognizing the importance of maintaining good health. Reducing mortality rates and improvements in life expectancy were the intended outcomes which were achievable by improving health infrastructure as well as spreading

---

[62] All the countries studied in this monograph are member countries of SAARC.

[63] The 30th World Health Assembly in May 1977 through resolution WHA30.43 decided that - "the main social target of governments and of WHO in the coming decades should be the attainment by all the citizens of the world by the year 2000 of a level of health that will permit them to lead a socially and economically productive life" (WHO, 1985, p. 1) which was translated as a mission to achieve "Health For All." This resolution considered health a basic human right and a world-wide social goal which is essential to the satisfaction of basic human needs and the quality of life.

the WHO's reach to all citizens. This was much greater a challenge for the South Asian region as it has historically suffered from a shortage of resources.

The data as retrieved from the World Bank database (Table 3.2 and Table 3.3) reveal that the governments of this region have not been able to spend as much as desired or as others per trends in world expenditure on health. The world expenditure was around 10% of the GDP which is more than 2.5 times what South Asia spends (3.72%) on health on average. In terms of specific countries, the Maldives and Afghanistan have increased government health expenditure, placing them far above world average. However, all other South Asian countries are spending much less on health of its citizens (Fig. 3.2). Regionally, East Asia and Pacific have only spent 6.77% on health, while Europe and Central Asia spent 9.34%, and South Africa spent 8.2% (Fig. 3.3). The estimates of current health expenditures include health-

Table 3.2 Current health expenditure as percentage of GDP

	2000	2005	2010	2015
Afghanistan	NA	9.95	8.57	10.30
Bangladesh	2.40	2.80	2.68	2.64
Bhutan	4.19	3.53	3.18	3.49
India	4.18	3.79	3.27	3.89
The Maldives	7.35	8.79	9.32	11.50
Nepal	3.57	4.51	4.97	6.15
Pakistan	3.09	2.92	2.60	2.69
Sri Lanka	4.14	3.78	2.97	2.97
South Asia	3.89	3.68	3.23	3.72
World	**8.60**	**9.33**	**9.53**	**9.90**

Source World development indicators, updated as on 14 November 2018 from http://databank. worldbank.org/data/source/world-development-indicators

Table 3.3 Current health expenditure as percentage of GDP

Region	2000	2005	2010	2015
South Asia	3.89	3.68	3.23	3.72
Sub-Saharan Africa	5.38	5.48	5.30	5.35
Middle East and North Africa	4.71	4.21	4.90	5.45
East Asia and Pacific	6.19	6.28	6.48	6.77
Latin America and Caribbean	6.09	6.52	6.87	7.39
Europe and Central Asia	7.79	8.45	9.03	9.34
Euro area	8.58	9.29	10.08	10.19
World	8.60	9.33	9.53	9.90

Source World development indicators, updated as on 14 November 2018 from http://databank. worldbank.org/data/source/world-development-indicators

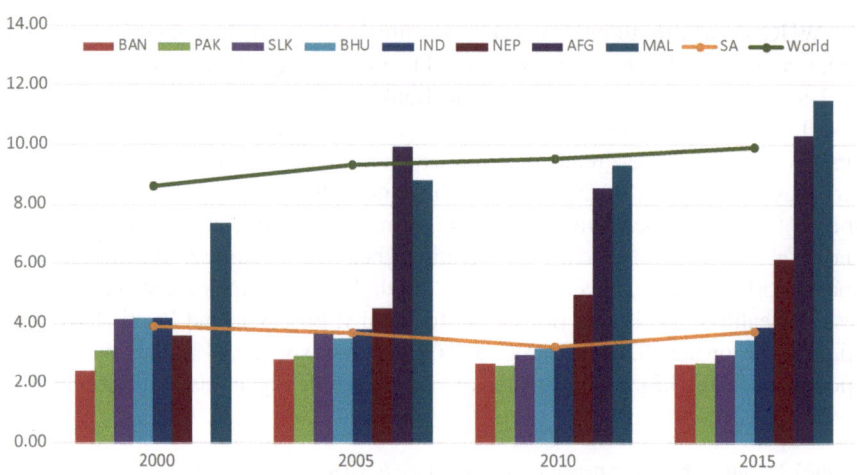

Fig. 3.2 Current health expenditure as percentage of GDP (South Asian region vis-a-vis world)

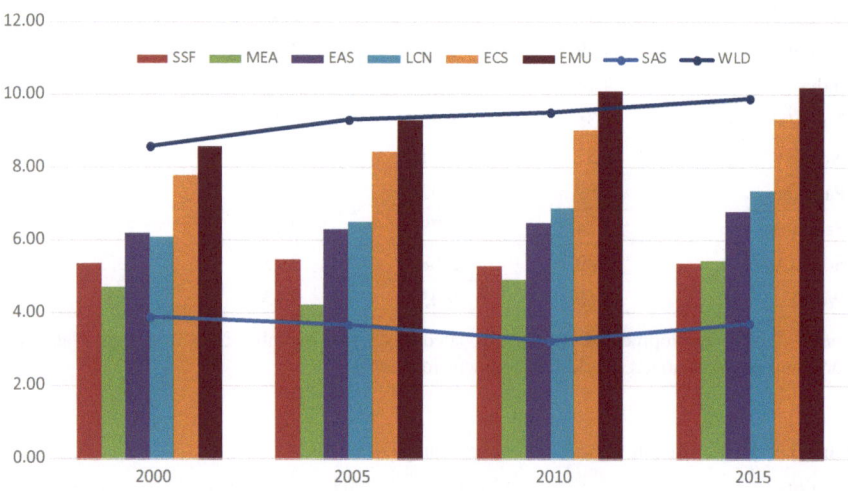

Fig. 3.3 Current health expenditure as percentage of GDP (world regions)

care goods and services consumed during each year. This indicator does not include capital health expenditures such as buildings, machinery, IT and stocks of vaccines for emergency or outbreaks.

As previously mentioned, government spending on health in the South Asian region is around one-third of world spending (Fig. 3.4). This low governmental spending is adversely affecting out-of-pocket health expenditure (share of out-of-pocket payments of total current health expenditures referring to spending on health directly out-of-pocket by households). This expenditure is estimated as the percentage of current health expenditure which was compared in the above section. The

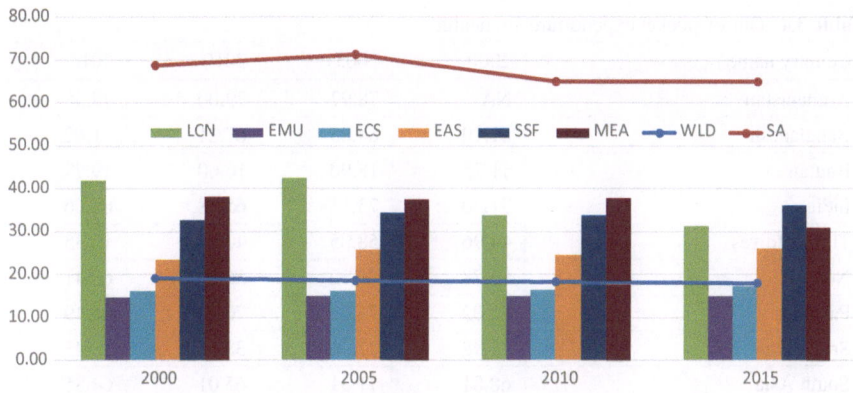

Fig. 3.4 Out-of-pocket expenditure on health (world region)

residents of South Asia spend the most on healthcare as compared to their counterparts living in other world regions, South Asian citizens are spending 3.5 times more than the world average. The households of South Asia spend roughly two times more than the households of Sub-Saharan Africa. In 2015, the household healthcare expenditure of South Asian households was more than four times that of European households (Table 3.4). Across all the South Asian countries, households in Bhutan consistently spent the least between 2000 and 2015. Households in the Maldives have halved their spending on health. Bhutan and the Maldives are currently close to the world average, whereas the households from all other countries of the region have been spending their might on health (Fig. 3.5).

As highlighted above the GDP spending pattern of South Asian countries on health has been much below the world standards except few countries. On the contrary out-of-pocket health expenditure has been on the rise across region with an exception of Bhutan. The participation of the private sector in health care has been very impressive in some parts of the region such as India, Sri Lanka, and Bangladesh. Though the private sector has helped improve health infrastructure in general, it has impacted the service attitude of medical professionals negatively. Profiteering has become the primary force to start hospitals and service attitude attached to the profession known for its nature of nobility is compromised at large. There are instances when corporate hospitals are found to be exploiting the patients for want of sustaining themselves.

Afghanistan has established an initiative to prevent poor health among the general population, achieve significant reductions in mortality in line with national targets (and SDGs), and to reduce impoverishment due to catastrophic health expenditure.[64] It also aims to make health facilities more accessible; keeping in mind quality, equitable distribution, and affordability for all. In order to improve the nutritional status of Afghanis, the government has committed to improving health financing, creating awareness among people about health and hygiene, and promoting a healthy

---

[64]The information has been obtained from the official website of the ministry of public health, Government of Afghanistan (http://moph.gov.af/en).

Table 3.4 Out-of-pocket expenditure on health

Country name	2000	2005	2010	2015
Afghanistan	NA	78.97	79.00	78.38
Bangladesh	61.10	64.85	67.21	71.82
Bhutan	11.25	18.90	16.60	19.79
India	71.70	73.15	65.18	65.06
The Maldives	44.96	58.05	40.68	16.35
Nepal	55.78	49.22	56.20	60.41
Pakistan	62.02	71.02	70.39	66.49
Sri Lanka	26.98	27.26	38.47	38.43
South Asia	68.81	71.31	65.01	64.85
Sub-Saharan Africa	32.67	34.46	33.80	36.25
Middle East and North Africa	38.22	37.65	37.87	30.82
Latin America and Caribbean	42.07	42.36	33.95	31.27
Euro area	14.77	14.95	14.94	15.01
Europe and Central Asia	16.10	16.17	16.50	17.35
East Asia and Pacific	23.47	25.78	24.69	26.11
World	19.21	18.53	18.33	18.15
South Asia	68.81	71.31	65.01	64.85

Source World development indicators last updated on 14 November 2018 from
http://databank.worldbank.org/data/source/world-development-indicators

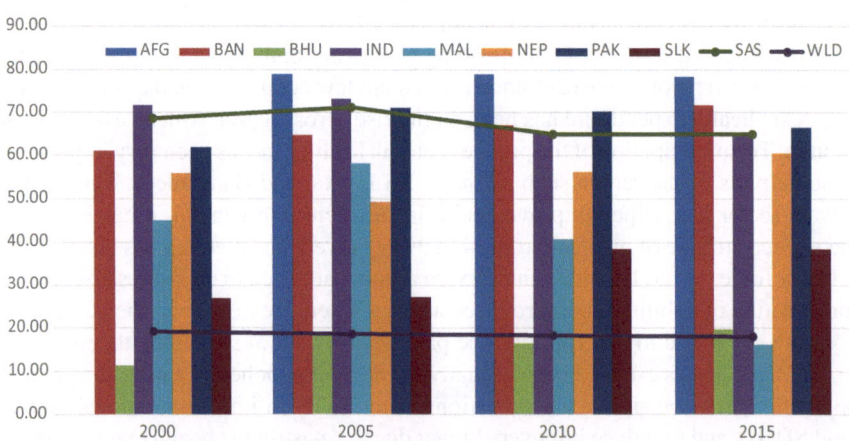

Fig. 3.5 Out-of-pocket expenditure on health (South Asian region)

environment. In 2011, Afghanistan published the National Health Policy[65] which ensured the establishment of a community clinic for every geographical area containing six thousand people, gender equity in health services per the One Health[66] approach, the right to access health information, and a health education unit in every *upazilla.*[67] The government has exemplified its commitment towards the "Health For All" campaign in these ways and provision for involvement of all stakeholders in improving health status. This commitment is expected to improve health parameters. Afghanistan government identifies NGOs and the private sector as equal partners who should play an active role in bettering the health of all citizens.

The World Bank signed a USD 100 million grant to Afghanistan in order to finance its System Enhancement for Health Action in Transition (SEHAT) program in May 2013.[68] Health has been one of the most important priorities on the government's planning agenda in the last decade. The SEHAT programs purpose is to expand the scope, quality, and coverage of health services; this is targeted especially towards the poor. SEHAT covered 21 provinces in the country out of 34, and is planned to extend to the other provinces as well—subject to availability of finances. Further, it identified three key components which are: 1. Sustaining and improving the basic package of health services and the essential package of hospital services; 2. Building the stewardship capacity of the ministry of public health and system development; and 3. Strengthening program management. Through all these initiatives Afghanistan has been able to improve public health indicators and reduce IMR. In November 2015, the ministry of public health published the National Health Policy 2015–2020. Major policy initiatives have been highlighted[69] as:

- Better balance of health and health care. Healthy lifestyles as a result of changing attitudes, perceptions, and practices while continuing to slow the incidence of communicable diseases and the maternal mortality and neonatal death rates.
- Improving access to, and quality of, basic health services working towards universal health coverage while improving tertiary care through private sector involvement and regulation.
- Changing governance and institutional functioning to achieve a more effective state ministry.

---

[65]The National Health Policy 2011 as available on http://www.mohfw.gov.bd/index.php?option=com_docman&task=doc_download&gid=1475&lang=enis in Bangla language. The key features have been highlighted.

[66]This is followed by the Bangladesh government which emphasises coordination among different ministries and departments related to public health and medical service.

[67]Second order after district.

[68]The information is obtained from the website of the World Bank available at: http://www.worldbank.org/en/news/press-release/2013/05/06/government-of-afghanistan-signs--100-million-grant-with-world-bank-to-improve-afghans-health-outcomes.

[69]See p. 6 of the report. The report is downloaded from the website of the ministry (http://moph.gov.af/Content/files/National%20health%20policy%202015-2020.pdf) retrieved on November 29, 2018.

- Creating a culture of responsibility, life-long learning, zero tolerance to corruption, merit-based appointments, performance evaluation, and more emphasis on the social determinants of health.
- Improved control over the quality of pharmaceuticals and food.

Drawing on Bhutan's development philosophy of GNH, the country has progressed steadily in terms of health indicators. Health is one of the prominent domains identified under GNH. In order to strengthen public health, in 2010[70] the government announced many initiatives including that the health sector would be opened to private investment and practices but would still be regulated by the government in terms of the quality of health services and human resources. The policy emphasizes that the participation of the private sector or of foreign companies and individuals shall not, under any circumstance, lead to the privatization of the public health services. In order to address the shortage of health personnel, it was decided that high-end private sector clinics and hospitals would be allowed to bring in as many expatriate doctors and nurses as necessary while still in keeping with the rules and regulations as prescribed by the Bhutan Health and Medical Council Act. The newly established pharmaceutical shops in the rural areas of Bhutan were given a five-year tax holiday during 2010–2015, and newly established, high-end private health services were eligible for a ten-year tax holiday. These policies have impacted health parameters positively and Bhutan is focusing its efforts on achieving the SDGs (Sustainable Development Goals) by their stated deadlines. Bhutan's 12th FYP (2018–2023) has prioritized access to quality health services as an important objective of the government.

India has been working to achieve its health targets and improve overall health conditions. It has made some improvements in health indicators, but these look small when compared with both other regions of the world as well as with other countries in South Asia. Healthcare is administratively managed by the both provincial governments in states and the national government at the center. All of the states are at liberty to make their own policies to improve the health of the residents, as long as these are within the overarching guidelines set forth by the central government of India.

In 2017, the Indian ministry of health and family welfare published its National Health Policy[71] which provided the desired direction for growth in the health sector. This policy is drafted in continuation of the government's commitment to health and the progress made thus far since the National Health Policy 2002. The broad goals of the 2017 policy are the attainment of the highest possible level of health and well-being for all, and universal access to good quality health care services, both of which should be achieved through increasing access, improving quality, and lowering the cost. The government has committed to achieving universal health coverage, reinforcing trust in the public health care system, and aligning the growth

---

[70] The information was obtained from The Economic Development Policy of the Kingdom of Bhutan 2010 which is available at the https://www.gnhc.gov.bt/en/wp-content/uploads/2017/05/EDP.pdf.
[71] See GOI (2017).

of the private health care sector with public health goals through attaining some of these targets:

- Increase life expectancy at birth from 67.5 years to 70 years by 2025.
- Establish regular tracking of Disability Adjusted Life Years Index as a measure of burden of disease and its trends by major categories by 2022.
- Reduction of Total Fertility Rate[72] to 2.1 (per woman) at national and sub-national level by 2025.
- Reduce under-five mortality to 23 by 2025, MMR from current levels to 100 by 2020, IMR to 28 by 2019, neo-natal mortality to 16, and still birth rate to "single digit" by 2025.
- To reduce the prevalence of blindness to 0.25 per 1000 by 2025 and disease burden by one-third from current levels.
- Increase utilization of public health facilities by 50% from current levels by 2025.
- Antenatal care coverage to be sustained above 90% and skilled attendance at birth to increase above 90% by 2025.
- More than 90% of newborns are fully immunized by one year of age by 2025.
- Meet the requirement of family planning[73] above 90% at national and sub national level by 2025.
- Relative reduction in the prevalence of current tobacco use by 15% by 2020 and 30% by 2025.
- Access to safe water and sanitation to all by 2020 (Swachh Bharat Mission).
- Increase in health expenditure by the government as a percentage of GDP from the existing 1.15–2.5% by 2025.
- Increase in the state sector health spending to more than 8% of their budget by 2020.
- Decrease in proportion of households facing catastrophic health expenditure from the current levels by 25%, by 2025.
- Ensure district-level electronic database of information on health system components by 2020.
- Strengthen the health surveillance system and establish registries for diseases of public health importance by 2020.
- Establish federated integrated health information architecture, Health Information Exchanges, and National Health Information Network by 2025.

India launched the National Health Mission (NHM) in 2013. For concentrating on urban populations, it has the National Urban Health Mission (NUHM) and for rural population, the National Rural Health Mission (NRHM)—which was initially

---

[72]Total Fertility Rate or TFR as it is used in demographic literature, is defined by the World Health Organization as—"the number of children born or likely to be born to a woman in her life time if she were subject to the prevailing rate of age specific fertility in the population". Retrieved from: http://www.searo.who.int/entity/health_situation_trends/data/chi/TFR/en/.

[73]India became the first country in the world to initiate family planning program in 1952 with the goal of lowering fertility and slowing the population growth rate (accessed from https://humdo.nhp.gov.in/about/national-fp-programme/).

launched in 2005. In 2013, NRHM got merged with the NHM. Using the above-mentioned health-centered targets, the government has initiated various programs to improving the health of its citizens. Some such programs are *Swasth Nagrik Abhiyan* (Healthy Citizen Campaign), *Swachh Bharat Abhiyan* (Clean India Campaign), *Yatri Suraksha* (a program to prevent deaths due to rail and road traffic accidents), *Nirbhaya Nari*,[74] *Pradhan Mantri Surakshit Matritva Abhiyan*,[75] etc. The government launched a new ministry on November 9, 2014 called the ministry of Ayurveda, Yoga and Naturopathy, Unani, Siddha and Homoeopathy (AYUSH).

Health parameters in the Maldives are the best in the region, as they have the highest life expectancy and the lowest IMR. The government is committed to providing equitable access to quality and affordable health services by practicing evidence-based decision-making in health policy formulation, extensive health care reform, and a nationally coordinated system for emergency medical services. The Maldives also promotes health awareness to all its citizens and encourages the practice of healthy lifestyles.

Poor health indicators have been a major concern for Nepal, which drove them to develop their Second Long-Term Health Plan (SLTHP) 1997–2017[76] in order to guide health sector development aimed towards improving the health of all citizens with a special emphasis on those whose health needs were not met thus far. The SLTHP made quality healthcare services available and accessible, and addressed disparities in the health sector. The plan also encouraged the involvement of women through gender sensitivity. The SLTHP also acted as a guiding force behind successive periodic and annual health plans. This plan provided a foundation on which appropriate action plans were drawn which reflected national health priorities that are affordable and consistent with available resources. However, Nepal's government expenditure is still too low to appropriately improve health indicators. This is partly due to the fact that Nepal is a traditionally poor nation with a minimal resource base, and it is more challenging for such nations to effectively implement sweeping reform. This is why these countries often ask for private partnerships who become development partners with the state to help shoulder the financial responsibility. Nepal through the SLTHP should coordinate efforts amongst public and private organizations and NGOs to work towards better health well-being for all of Nepal. It also hoped to provide an appropriate number of technically competent staff with a sense of social responsibility to improve the quality of healthcare services-staff who are willing to serve throughout the country, particularly in under-served and remote areas. The SLTHP also expected to increase efficiency and effectiveness of the healthcare system by improving overall management of public health care sector.

In quantitative terms, the SLTHP targeted to reduce: IMR to 34.4 (per 1000 live births), under-five mortality rate to 62.5 (per 1000), total fertility rate to 3.05 (per woman), crude birth rate to 26.6 (per 1000), crude death rate to 6 (per 1000), maternal

---

[74]This is a hindi term, if translated in English it means—action against gender violence.

[75]This is a hindi term, if translated in English it means—Prime Minister safe maternity campaign.

[76]The information regarding SLTHP is obtained from the department's website which is available at: dohs.gov.np/wp-content/uploads/2014/04/2nd-Long-Term-Health-Plan.docx.

Table 3.5 Target of SLTHP[a] and achievement

Health indicator	Unit	Target 2017	Achieved 2016 (See Ministry of Health, Nepal (2017). Accessed from https://phpnepal. org.np/publication/ current-issue/recently- released/195-full-report- of-nepal-demographic- and-health-survey-ndhs- 2016)
IMR	Per '000 live births	34.4	32
Under-5 mortality rate	Per '000	62.5	39
Total fertility rate	Per woman	3.05	2.3
Crude birth rate	Per '000	26.6	22
Maternal mortality rate	Per hundred '000 births	250	239
Contraceptive prevalence rate	Percent	58.2	53

[a]Second Long-Term Health Plan (SLTHP)

mortality rate to 250 (per hundred thousand births), the percentage of iron-deficiency anemia among pregnant women to 15%. It hoped to increase: life expectancy to 68.7 years, the contraceptive prevalence rate to 58.2%, the percentage of deliveries attended by trained personnel to 95%, pregnant women attending a minimum of four antenatal visits to 80%, the percentage of women of child-bearing age (15–44) who receive tetanus toxoid (TT2) to 90%, and total health expenditures to 10% of total government expenditures by 2017. It hoped to also have essential healthcare services in the districts available to 90% of the population living within a 30 min travel time of available facilities and to equip 100% of facilities with full staff in order to deliver essential healthcare services. According to the Nepal Demographic Health Survey 2016, it had achieved most of these targets (Table 3.5).

Pakistan has some of the worst health parameters in the South Asian region. The government in Pakistan launched its national health policy in 2016, called the National Health Vision after failing to have any health policy in place for the previous 15 years.[77] This made healthcare policies uniform across the country. The National Health Vision (2016–2025)[78] identifies the health-related challenges that Pakistan has faced in past years and states that universal health coverage is one of the ultimate

---

[77]As per report in *Dawn*—national daily newspaper appeared on 31st Aug 2016—https://www. dawn.com/news/1281107 (retrieved on 14 Sept 2018).

[78]The National Health Vision document is available at http://www.nationalplanningcycles.org/ sites/default/files/planning_cycle_repository/pakistan/national_health_vision_2016-25_30-08- 2016.pdf.

goals of the ministry of national health services, regulation, and coordination in Pakistan. The vision statement of the National Health Vision[79] reads as:

> To improve the health of all Pakistanis, particularly women and children, through universal access to affordable quality essential health services, and delivered through resilient and responsive health system, ready to attain Sustainable Development Goals and fulfill its other global health responsibilities. (p. 3)

The national vision plan details eight thematic pillars that should guide overall health policy which are the provision of financing, service delivery, human resources, information system, governance, essential medicines and technology, cross sectoral linkages, and global health responsibilities. It is put forth in order to improve health, responsiveness, social protection, and efficiency. The plan's goals are improving the coverage and functionality of primary and promotive health services, enforcing public health laws, and developing effective linkages with the private sector in service delivery. The National Health Vision is very promising and highlights the government's concerns involving healthcare. It has helped Pakistan to improve health parameters which has been discussed in Chap. 2.

Sri Lanka has been an outstanding country in terms of its health indicators. It is the only country in South Asia which is ranked among the high human development countries in the HDI. Sri Lanka's National Health Policy 2016–2025[80] issued by the ministry of health, nutrition, and indigenous medicine, provides the framework for its overall health improvement plan over a 10-year period. The guiding principles as stated in the policy focus on a patient and people centric approach that focuses on universal health coverage through equitable access, and distribution of quality and economical services to all patients. The major targets of the policy are:

- To strengthen surveillance of food and water borne diseases.
- To eliminate human rabies by 2020.
- To maintain zero transmission of Malaria and Filariasis.
- To improve the health status of the plantation community by reducing the disparity that exists between the people residing in plantation areas and the other regions of the country.
- To establish an anti-microbial stewardship program in all hospitals.
- To ensure the efficient and effective supply of quality medical items to relevant health institutions.
- To ensure healthy ageing with multi sectoral collaboration.
- To ensure patient's rights, public confidence, and patient/client satisfaction at all public and private health institutions.
- To regulate the private health sector to ensure quality service and financial risk protection for the patients.
- To strengthen regulation regarding the prices of medicinal drugs and devices.

---

[79]Ibid.

[80]Retrieved on September 18, 2019 from http://www.health.gov.lk/moh_final/english/public/ elfinder/files/publications/policiesUpto2016/policiesForPublicOpinion/NHP2016-2025draft.pdf.

- To establish a National Health Performance Monitoring System to track the health system's performance.
- To collaborate with international donor agencies in improving the health status of Sri Lankans as per this National Health Policy.

The government has also prepared a strategic master plan on these aspects in order to achieve health goals and improve the well-being of Sri Lankans.

Though not the case for outliers such as Sri Lanka or the Maldives, the region as a whole has not been able to maintain an acceptable standard of health conditions. The amount of government health expenditure is much lower than in other world regions. In the majority of South Asia, the health sector has been privatized which has demonstrated its own pros and cons. Individual spending on health is on the rise and the rate in South Asia is one of the highest across world. Though the prevalence of some chronic diseases like malaria, cholera, and polio have been reduced in the region, a rise in cases related to non-communicable diseases like cardiovascular diseases, diabetes, and cancer has been observed. The countries in the region must devise ways to more effectively manage future health concerns so that the physical well-being of people is assured.

3.5 Initiatives to Improve Governance

Good governance has been a challenge and often a casualty for all of South Asia. As a result, the absence of good governance has negatively affected the progress of the region. Endowed with rich natural resources and diversity, the region has failed to capitalize on these strengths due to poor governance practices. Poor compliance levels, corrupt practices, and an indifferent attitude in the responsible officers have resulted in submissive mindset among the masses. Corruption is prevalent in South Asia and as such has seeped into the psyche of the majority of the residents of the region. Bhutan is an exceptional country with a strong democratic system of government, which it has had for around a decade. However, even there, corruption has been one of the significant issues plaguing general elections as political parties often face allegations of corruption by the members of ruling government. Across South Asia, general elections are waged on issues concerning poor governance and corruption. As discussed in Chap. 2, Afghanistan, Pakistan, Bangladesh, and Nepal are the most affected countries. India and Sri Lanka face a similar level of corruption and ineffective governance. Conditions in the Maldives are worsening.

Local governance is the key to building confidence by involving citizens at the ground level. In Afghanistan local governance was largely absent until 2017, when the independent electoral commission announced its long-delayed elections which were to assure democratic reform in the country. The local councils of the independent directorate of local governance, have drafted law which is aimed at improving local governance in Afghanistan. The United States Agency for International Development (USAID) supports Afghanistan governmental reform[81] which is working to improve its governance through boosting transparency and accountability, making government processes more efficient, improving public outreach, and strengthening linkages between central and sub-national levels of government. The USAID is a governance partner with Afghanistan's state government and helps with delivering essential services at a local level, community engagement, and establishing well-governed, fiscally sound institutions. The United Nations Development Programme (UNDP) is also helping Afghanistan improve parliamentary transparency and accountability through increased media access to parliamentary activities.

The UNDP also supports the implementation of governance reforms in Pakistan.[82] It has suggested strong civil service reforms based on an in-depth study on areas of government recruitment, training, institutional structures, compensation, and performance management. With the support of UNDP, a citizen perception survey was introduced as a part of the Open Government Initiative,[83] which is the first ever survey of its kind in Pakistan.

Bangladesh's Quarterly Development Update (October–December 2017)[84] reports that with the digitalization of its public administration, the Bangladesh government has been able to raise transparency and curb bureaucratic inefficiencies. The government has increased discipline in public financial management and improved service delivery. Quasi-independent bodies, such as the Human Rights Commission and the Right to Information Commission, have been established to register the grievances of the citizenry. The 7th FYP (2016–2020) and Vision 2021 reflect areas of good governance and reforms. The quarterly update of the last quarter of 2017 states that Bangladesh has not been able to meet the set governance targets and thus more reforms are required. The Country Assistance Strategy of the World Bank has identified governance as the fourth pillar of priority and offered support to help Bangladesh improve the quality of governance.

The UNDP is working very closely with Nepal's government to help it build better systems to improve governance. It is focusing on improving the process, mechanism, and outcome for better governance. In this context, the process refers to the quality of participation necessary to ensure that political, social, and economic priorities are based on a broad consensus in society and that the voices of the excluded, poorest, and most vulnerable, are heard in decision-making. The mechanism refers to inclusion of transparent and democratic institutions necessary for effective governance. The outcome of good governance is expected to include peaceful, stable, and resilient societies, where services are delivered and reflect the needs of communities, including

---

[81] Accessed from https://www.usaid.gov/afghanistan/democracy-governance.

[82] Accessed from http://www.pk.undp.org/content/pakistan/en/home/operations/projects/democratic_governance/governance-reforms-and-innovation-.html.

[83] Accessed from https://www.undp.org/content/dam/pakistan/docs/Project%20Briefs/April2017/DGU/Project%20brief%20-%20Governance%20Reforms%20and%20Innovation.pdf.

[84] Accessed from http://www.bd.undp.org/content/dam/bangladesh/docs/Publications/Pub-2018/Bangladesh%20Quarterly%20Development%20Update.pdf.

the voices of the most vulnerable and marginalized.[85] The UNDP is involved in advocating, advising, fostering impartial spaces for dialogue, achieving consensus, and building institutions with the ultimate goal of bringing effective and equitable delivery of service to citizens and reinforcing the rule of law and citizen security.

India's current government, which was first elected in 2014 and re-elected in 2019 in recently held general elections, prioritized improving governance and curbing corruption with a zero-tolerance policy.[86] Toward these goals, India demonetized currency notes of INR 500 and INR 1000 denominations in 2016 trying to curb corruption, unearth black (unaccounted) money, and uproot terrorism. Terrorism is widely believed to be funded by counterfeit currency notes of INR 500 and INR 1000. The government announced the double tax avoidance treaty with Mauritius, Cyprus, and Singapore; and signed an agreement to exchange real time information with Switzerland, where illegal money is frequently deposited by corrupt politicians and business people. The Insolvency and Bankruptcy Code of 2016 is considered one of most important economic reforms in India. The code provides a one-stop solution for resolving insolvencies which were previously taking a long time to process. The clauses of the code help protecting the interests of small investors and are targeted towards reduction in corrupt practices. The Benami Transactions (Prohibition) Amendment Act of 2016 has laid the foundation for a future corruption-free India. The Whistle Blower's Protection Act, 2011 and the Prevention of Corruption Act, 1988 were amended to safeguard the interest of whistle blowers.

The use of technology in the delivery of government services has been enhanced through the Digital India program, which helped make transactions formal, transparent, and efficient, and has reduced bureaucratic procedures. The MyGov portal and app is a landmark government initiative to help ensure good governance and engage with citizens. The government has taken action against more than two hundred thousand companies suspected of money laundering. When it comes to good governance, much depends on commitment levels. The government in India seems to have created an eco-system which is taking action against corruption thus conveying a strong positive message to citizens.

The countries of the South Asian region have shown their commitment to improve HWB through the various initiatives, policies, and programs detailed in this chapter. Despite the multifaceted nature of the problems facing South Asia, the region as a whole has largely been able to implement effective policies and has invested their resources in increasing development. Poverty levels have improved, GDP per capita is increasing, access to education has expanded, and revised health policies are in place. Though access to education has improved well, improvement in quality of education is much needed. State allocations for health have been abysmally low as compared to world standards, resulting in the proliferation of private hospitals which are beyond the reach of the poor population. Though education is one of the focus

---

[85] Accessed   from   http://www.np.undp.org/content/nepal/en/home/democratic-governance/in-depth.html.

[86] Accessed from http://pibarchive.nic.in/ndagov/Initiatives.aspx.

areas of public policy, yet the allocation out of GDP expenditure on education is not as expected and needs attention of policy makers. Overall when we look at all the indicators, the biggest concern has been poor governance across region. Jamil, Askvik, and Dhakal (2013) state:

> Different reforms, institutional changes and creation of new acts, policies, and new organizations have been tried to streamline public administration and governance mechanisms both at the central and local levels. In spite of many experiments and innovative efforts, governance thus far has remained weak, unresponsive to citizen needs, centralized, rigid, non-transparent, and unaccountable. (p. 15)

In order to improve governance practices in the whole South Asian region, transparency in transactions and good intent are required at all levels of governance, which requires committed efforts to improving HWB in South Asia.

References

Ahsan, M. (2003). An analytical review of Pakistan's educational policies and plans. *Research Papers in Education, 18*(3), 259–280. https://doi.org/10.1080/0267152032000107329.

Bandara, J. S. (2009). *Trade and poverty in South Asia: An interpretive survey.* Discussion Paper No. 2009-09. Griffith Business School, Economics.

Banks, C. (1995). *Rumi—Selected Poems.* London: Penguin Classics.

Bhattarai, K. (2011). Trade, growth and poverty in South Asia. In R. Jha (Ed.), *Routledge handbook of South Asian economics* (pp. 258–276). New york: Routledge.

Dundar, H., Beteille, T., Riboud, M., & Deolalikar, A. (2014). *Student learning in South Asia: Challenges, opportunities and policy priorities.* Washington DC: The World Bank. https://doi.org/10.1596/978-1-4648-0160-0.

GOI. (2017). *National health policy 2017.* New Delhi, India: Ministry of Health and Family Welfare, Government of India. Retrieved from http://cdsco.nic.in/writereaddata/National-Health-Policy.pdf.

Jamil, I., Askvik, S., & Dhakal, T. N. (2013). Understanding governance in South Asia. In I. Jamil, S. Askvik, & T. N. Dhakal (Eds.), *In search of better governance in South Asia and beyond, public administration, governance and globalization* (pp. 13–35). New York: Springer.

Jha, R. (2011). Fiscal policies and challenges in South Asia. In R. Jha (Ed.), *Routledge handbook of South Asian economics* (pp. 171–181). New York: Routledge.

Khandker, S. R., Khalily, M. A. B., & Samad, H. A. (2016). *Beyond ending poverty—The dynamics of microfinance in Bangladesh.* Washington, D.C.: World Bank. https://doi.org/10.1596/978-1-4648-0894-4.

Kinga, S. (2009). *Kingship and democracy—A biography of the Bhutanese state.* Thimphu: Ministry of Education, Royal Government of Bhutan.

Langer, A., Stewart, F., & Venugopal, R. (Eds.). (2012). *Horizontal inequalities and post-conflict development.* New York: Palgrave Macmillan. https://doi.org/10.1057/9780230348622.

Malak, M. (2013). Inclusive education reform in Bangladesh: Pre-service teachers' responses to include students with special educational needs in regular classrooms. *International Journal of Instruction, 6*(1), 195–214. Retrieved from https://files.eric.ed.gov/fulltext/ED539903.pdf.

Martin, R., Béteille, T., Li, Y., Mitra, P. K., & Newman, J. L. (2015). *Addressing inequality in South Asia.* Washington, DC: International Bank for Reconstruction and Development/The World Bank.

Ministry of Health, Nepal. (2017). *Nepal demographic and health survey 2016.* Kathmandu: United States Agency for International Development.

Muqtada, M. (1987). Special employment schemes in rural Bangladesh: Issues and perspective. *Philippine Review of Economics, 24*(3/4), 323–386.

Planning Commission. (1999). *Bhutan 2020: A vision for peace, prosperityand happiness. Part II*. Thimphu: Royal Government of Bhutan. Retrieved from http://www.gnhc.gov.bt/wp-content/uploads/2011/05/Bhutan2020_2.pdf.

PPD. (2018). *32nd education policy guidelines and instructions 2018*. Thimphu: Policy and Planning Division, Ministry of Education, Royal government of Bhutan.

Pursell, G. (2011). Trade policies in South Asia. In R. Jha (Ed.), *Routledge handbook of South Asian economics* (pp. 219–237). New York: Routledge.

Sgroi, D., Hills, T., O'Donnell, G., Oswald, A., & Proto, E. (2017). In K. Brandon (Ed.), *Understanding happiness: A CAGE policy report*. London: The Social Market Foundation.

WHO. (1985). *Handbook of resolutions and decisions of the world health assembly and the executive board. Volume II, 1973–1984*. Geneva: World Health Organization. Accessed from: http://apps.who.int/iris/bitstream/10665/79012/12/9241652063_Vol2.pdf.

World Bank. (2013). *Achieving learning for all*. Washington, DC: The World Bank. Accessed from http://www.worldbank.org/content/dam/Worldbank/Feature%20Story/Education/1317335_HDN_Education_Overview.pdf.

Zepeda, E., McDonald, S., Panda, M., Kumar, G., & Sapkota, C. (2013). *Employing India: Guaranteeing jobs for the rural poor*. Washington, DC: Carnegie Endowment for International Peace.

Chapter 4
Human Well-Being Policy and Discussion

Prajasukhe sukham ragyaha prajaanam tu hite hitam,
Naatmapriyyam hitam ragyaha prajaanam tu hitam priyam.
[In the happiness of his subjects lies his happiness; in their
welfare his welfare; whatever pleases himself he shall not
consider as good, but whatever pleases his subjects he shall
consider as good.]
[Kautilya][a]

Abstract The world has evolved in speed and space, in wealth and health, in knowledge and wisdom, and the process is continuous. These changes have expanded the horizon of our thinking and raised our expectations of society, government, and our fellow man. South Asia is no exception to this trend. There are more visible democracies, there are larger and taller buildings than ever, the average lifespan has increased, there are more schools and hospitals, people are more connected in this digital age, and more people are living above the poverty line. These changes impart a general feeling that the present is a better and happier time to live than any other time in history. This mindset is what has to be studied in order to determine whether the visible progress has truly been translated into better human well-being or not. This chapter examines the input (Chap. 3) and outcome (Chap. 2) concerning given indicators and the narrative they create. This chapter gives a detailed discussion on economic progress and policy; health and education; and politics and governance. Changes as they have occurred are narrated through published reports and research which help the reader to understand the region, indicators, and the larger story of South Asia.

Keywords Human well-being · South Asia · Public policy · GDP · Health · Education · Governance · Poverty

4.1 Introduction

Human well-being is a construct evolved from the philosophy of living well—mentally, physically, socially, and spiritually. Individuals tend to perform acts that (they

---

[a]see Rangarajan 1992, p. 125.

© Springer Nature Switzerland AG 2020
V. K. Shrotryia, *Human Well-Being and Policy in South Asia*, Human Well-Being
Research and Policy Making, https://doi.org/10.1007/978-3-030-33270-9_4

think) will provide them satisfaction and lead towards improving their state of "living well". Fulfillment of human needs and having a positive living environment, contributes towards an assurance of 'living well' or leading a good life. Physical facilities enhance mental satisfaction and help in realizing human potential by exploring different possibilities and choices. Being able to use physical facilities further require resources of different kind—good health, knowledge and ability, money, a conducive eco-system, and enabling infrastructure. These resources are internal as well as external, they are possessions as well as acquisitions. Available literature on well-being, happiness, and quality of life directly or indirectly revolves around this philosophy of living well. Hedonism, eudemonism, utilitarianism, consequentialism, and the like '-isms' defend the use of a construct named as HWB. The whole idea of HWB, happiness, and living well spans the 'compulsion' to 'choice' continuum.

The state (or government) plans and makes effective policies for the well-being of its citizens by providing opportunities to earn a living, investing in human capital by provision of health and education, and building facilitating physical infrastructure. These policies, when implemented successfully, should reap fruits such as economic progress, improved health, increased education, and empowered citizens. The responsibility to look after social welfare is shared by four core institutions—the state, the market, the family, and the civil society (Estes & Zhou, 2014). Policy formulation and its implementation are mediated as well as moderated by the effectiveness of the system involved in implementation. Mediation explains process between policy creation and its execution. Moderation measures the effectiveness of policy as low or high and may be, in numbers or degree. The effectiveness of the system is assured by the state through strong governance measures. However sound policies are, if not implemented effectively, they would fail to affect the intended population. Smith (1984) so succinctly puts it in one of his classics, *The Theory of Moral Sentiments*, written nearly three centuries years ago:

> In what constitutes the real happiness of human life … In ease of body and peace of mind, all the different ranks of life are nearly upon a level, and the beggar, who suns himself by the side of the highway, possesses that security which kings are fighting for. … The same principle, the same love of system, the same regard to the beauty of order, of art and contrivance, frequently serves to recommend those institutions which tend to promote the public welfare. When a patriot exerts himself for the improvement of any part of the public police, his conduct does not always arise from pure sympathy with the happiness of those who are to reap the benefit of it. (p. 185)

The state, through its policy, and the monarch, through their charter, only can claim to look after the welfare of its citizens. It has the responsibility to efficiently manage resources through equitable distribution for the good of the citizens.

Earlier chapters have analyzed and narrated the outcome of indicators (Chap. 2) and input indicators (Chap. 3). In this chapter, comparisons are made and discussed at length to explain the gaps between input and outcome (if any), good practices, trends, and expectations in order to provide a guide for future policy direction. The purpose of this book is to urge policymakers to reexamine their priorities (if required), and to provide good practices to be followed further or expose bad practices to be revised and discontinued (whatever necessary).

4.2 Poverty, Problems and Progress—Towards Human Well-Being in South Asia

It is quite encouraging to know that "societies worldwide have made enormous progress in improving the socioeconomic conditions for large groups of people over the last century. Just in the last 20 years, more than 1.2 billion people have been lifted out of poverty" (World Bank, 2015a). As Nobel Laureate Angus Deaton labels this achievement "the great escape" or "the story of mankind's escaping from deprivation and early death, of how people have managed to make their lives better, and led the way for others to follow" (Deaton, 2013, p. ix).[1] The driving force behind this progress has been the ability of deprived people to reach a minimum level of subsistence. Rosling (2018) provides an exceptional account of progress the world has made over the last decades which in general people perceive otherwise. The accomplishments of the South Asian region in the area of economic growth (income) is much better as compared to improvements in health, education, and subjective well-being, all of which are modest when compared with the gains attained in the same areas by other regions of the world. As reported in the preliminary report of OPHI (2018, p. x), India has been able to cut its poverty rate from 55 to 28% (over 270 million people) in 10 years' time, from June 2005 to June 2015. Which is similar to China's achievement over a decade ago.

Poor health is both a consequence and a cause of poverty. Poverty is still persistent in most of the countries in South Asia. Though there has been positive and significant improvement, and fewer people are living in extreme poverty, disparities are on rise. Increased inequality should not be the price of economic growth. But economic theories have proved that inequality is a byproduct of economic growth. Economists and policy makers have raised their concern and models are being suggested to reduce inequalities so that fruits of economic growth are distributed appropriately. De Neve and Powdthavee (2016) studied data from the Gallup World Poll and the World Top Income Database and reported that the more income is concentrated in the hands of a few, the more likely individuals are to report lower levels of life satisfaction and more negative daily emotional experiences. Hence the policies of a developing country should be designed to promote economic growth in such a way that concentration of wealth in a few hands is avoided. Gandhi stated that "the earth has enough to satisfy everybody's need but not anybody's greed." Gandhi's thinking is very relevant to HWB and happiness, as it provides long-term sustainable solutions instead of short-term gains (Shrotryia, 2005). His life was a message in itself.

Most South Asian countries have made considerable progress in human development over the last few decades; but despite this they have not been able to allocate appropriate resources to health and education. Investment in people through the provision of good health and education needs to be a priority for developing nations in order to assure better HWB. South Asia must be able to learn from the experience of

---

[1] As cited in World Bank (2017, p. 40).

a country which is ranked significantly higher in terms of human development. For example:

> When Sweden made schooling compulsory for all children in 1842, its GDP per capita (USD 926) was lower than the current GDP per capita of all the countries in South Asia. So, high national income is not a prerequisite for taking the first steps towards broad-based investment in providing basic social services. Investment in public services precedes growth. (UNDP, 2014, p. 87)

Low school attendance and poor educational infrastructure in general have been major problems and a challenge for the region as state investments in this area have been much lower as compared to other regions. Sri Lanka and the Maldives, both have better well-being indicators as compared to other South Asian countries. Afghanistan has suffered terribly during the last few decades and is considered one of the poorest and most corrupt countries in the world. Its GDP is largely dependent on aid and remittances from Afghans abroad—much of the budget allocation comes from abroad and nearly half of all government money is spent on security. The Kabul bank scandal that exploded between 2010 and 2013 almost caused state bankruptcy. The Afghani national budget for 2018 contains a myriad of items that were purposefully omitted or concealed. Afghanistan is primarily dealing with two key problems—one, the amount of international money coming into the country has declined and is expected to decline further in coming year; two, vulnerability to corruption is harming budget process. Formulating the national budget has been a process which—in the words of Integrity Watch Afghanistan—"has been riddled with incompetence, corruption, and collusion among the Executive and the National Assembly in the last decade".[2] In this light, it is remarkable that things are currently changing for good. Among all South Asian countries, it is Afghan households which spend highest on health.

Although South Asia is still predominately rural, 5% of the population moved from rural to urban areas between 1990 and 2010.[3] Studies show that unemployed people report lower levels of happiness and life satisfaction than their employed counterparts (Blanchflower & Oswald, 2011; Winkelmann & Winkelmann, 1998), however, farmers in South Asia report even lower levels of life satisfaction than the unemployed. Self-employed and wage earners of this region report similar levels of life satisfaction. Overall, only Sub-Saharan African populations report lower levels of life satisfaction than South Asian populations (World Bank, 2012). In recent years, South Asia has become the fastest growing region of the world, with per capita GDP growth rapidly accelerating in the last two decades.

Although the quality of life of the people in South Asia has improved over recent decades, it still lags significantly behind that of other world regions. This multilingual, multi-religion, multiethnic, and multicultural region is the poorest, most illiterate, most malnourished, and least gender-sensitive region in the world. Though women

---

[2]Accessed from https://www.afghanistan-analysts.org/the-2018-afghan-national-budget-confronting-hard-realities-by-accelerating-reforms/ on November 28, 2011.

[3]In 1990, 75.1% of the South Asian population resided in rural areas; in 2000, the number dropped to 72.6% and in 2010, to 69.9% (Trading Economics, 2015).

have started participating in the workforce—and discussions on female empower-ment is on the political and social agenda for policy and practice—the conditions of women have not materially improved as compared to other regions of the world. A field study (Datta, 2013) conducted in India (Awadh plains and Uttarakhand region) observed that the majority of women tend to have lower levels of well-being because they are less valued within the household and the community as their male counter-parts.

Considerable resources are channeled into military budgets rather than into human development. Interestingly in the case of India during 2018 and 2019, the defense allocation out of GDP has gone down to 1.56% which is its lowest since 1962. This is a positive indicator for the whole region, though the region still experiences repeated border hostilities; recurrent internal, communal, and ethnic conflicts; and outbreaks of violence in different areas which all effect quality of life. In general, all the countries of the region have experienced internal conflict in the last two decades, and the resulting casualties have outnumbered those from interstate conflicts.

Except for large-scale initiatives undertaken in South Asia by the SAARC and the United Nation's Millennium Development Campaign, few global initiatives—apart from projects targeted at local villages and communities—are designed to help raise the low levels of social development and well-being that have existed for decades. Even recent, sometimes dramatic, increases in the per capita income level have not succeeded in lifting South Asian populations to higher levels of social achievement.

The lag in well-being can be traced to the region's continued high rates of popula-tion increase; the existence—despite its illegality—of the caste system; the inferior status conferred to women; and, more existentially, the philosophies of the region that teach acceptance of one's place in society rather than social achievement and upwards social mobility. South Asia has the comparatively lowest female participa-tion rate in the labor force, which reflects on low status awarded to women in the region. In India and Pakistan, only 25–27% of women are in the labor force when they constitute around 48.3% of the population. Those who do work generally do so in less economically productive sectors and in occupations with potentially lower on-the-job learning opportunities (World Bank, 2018, p. 96).

The Georgetown Institute for Women, Peace and Security (GIWPS) published Women, Peace and Security Index 2017–2018. A primary goal of the index is to accelerate progress on both the international Women, Peace and Security agenda and the Sustainable Development Goals, bringing partners together around an agenda for women's inclusion, justice, and security. (GIWPS, 2017, p. viii). The index has drawn attention of policymakers, civil society, development agencies and academics through its inclusive approach towards providing valuable insights into issues con-cerning women and society. The composite index of 153 countries is based on gen-der, development, peace and indices covering three basic dimensions of well-being–inclusion (economic, social, political); justice (formal laws and informal discrim-ination); and security (at the family, community, and societal levels). It primarily focuses on the conditions of women across different countries and this index has covered around 98% of the world's population. The position of the South Asian countries is shown in Table 4.1 providing average index ratings and rank order in the world. It depicts the conditions of women in Afghanistan as worst in the world (and in South Asia as well) (Fig. 4.1) and that of Nepal as best in South Asia.

Several initiatives have tried to remedy this, such as the World Bank who financed the vocational training of 4400 young women leading to their employment and economic independence.[4] Even accounting for such initiatives and the minimal improvements that the region has experienced, more is needed in order to affect lasting change. Certainly, all of these factors contribute to the region's pattern of social stagnation even as progress is made in one or more critical social indicators.

If both paid and unpaid work is considered, women work more hours than men across the globe. Women spend a significant amount of their time performing unpaid jobs, much more so than men, which is not taken into account for calculation of GDP as argued by Burchardt (2013). A recent survey[5] shows that Latin Americans work the most hours a day (8.3 h for women as against 7.7 h for men), followed by the population in South Asia (7.7 h for women and 6.8 h for men). In South Asia, women's daily average time spent on unpaid work is 6.5 times that of men. And men in South Asia work less than an hour a day for unpaid job, which is least among all men in the world. Promisingly, ILO's India Wage Report[6] says that women's employment has

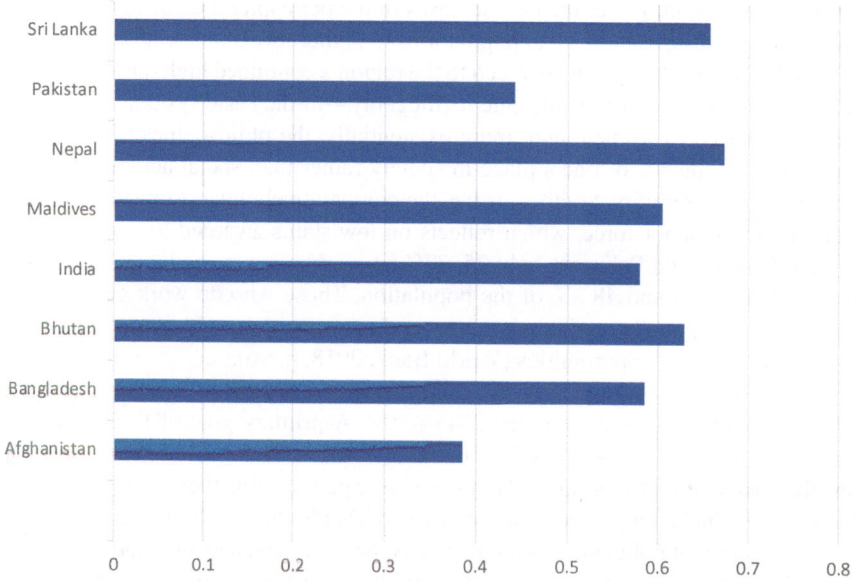

Fig. 4.1 Women, peace, and security index 2017

[4] See https://www.worldbank.org/en/region/sar/overview#3 as updated on July 16, 2018.

[5] See   https://sowf.men-care.org/wp-content/uploads/sites/4/2017/06/PRO17004_REPORT-Post-print-June9-WEB-3.pdf accessed on June 24, 2018.

[6] See   https://www.ilo.org/wcmsp5/groups/public/---asia/---ro-bangkok/---sro-new_delhi/documents/publication/wcms_638305.pdf accessed on September13, 2018.

Table 4.1 Women, peace, and security index 2017

Country	Average index rating	World rank ($n = 153$)
Afghanistan	0.385	152
Bangladesh	0.585	127
Bhutan	0.628	108
India	0.58	131
The Maldives	0.605	120
Nepal	0.672	85
Pakistan	0.441	150
Sri Lanka	0.656	97

Source Women, Peace, and Security Index, 2017, Georgetown Institute for Women, Peace and Security: Washington DC. Accessed from https://giwps.georgetown.edu/the-index/ on Aug 18, 2018

recently risen much faster than men's which has narrowed the gender wage gap. Women organizations in Afghanistan, with support from international donors and NGOs have made concerted lobbying efforts and mobilized support of the members of parliament and state officials to influence the drafting of a new law for ending violence against women. This law is known as Elimination of Violence Against Women or EVAW that criminalized gender violence for the first time in the history of Afghanistan. This law came into force in 2013 which is actively being used by activists for litigation and fighting for gender parity (Larson, 2016). This is historic considering the typical governance that has prevailed in Afghanistan.

South Asia as a region has historically enjoyed a wealthy reputation, prosperous living styles, and much better general HWB as compared to its contemporary counterparts. These inducements drove Alexander to invade in 326 BC through Takshila in the Indian subcontinent (presently in Pakistan) and the British to enter in 1600 AD through the port in Surat (presently in the state of Gujarat, India). Von (2007) described the region as:

> In the beginning, there were two nations. One was a vast, mighty and magnificent empire, brilliantly organized and culturally unified, which dominated a massive swath of the earth. The other was an undeveloped, semi-feudal realm, driven by religious factionalism and barely able to feed its illiterate, diseased and stinking masses. The first nation was India. The second was England. The year was 1577, and the Mughal emperors were in the process of uniting India. (p. 11)

Though these sentences describe India, they were written when India included Bangladesh and Pakistan. These sentences provide a historical perspective on the general well-being of the population of this region. Further, Bose and Jalal (2004) mention that:

> Between 1870 and 1914 India's export surplus was critical for Britain's balance of payments. Growing protectionism in continental Europe and America made it difficult for Britain to sell its manufactured goods while being dependent on importing a broad range of their agricultural commodities. It was in this context that Indian raw material exports to America

and continental Europe proved vital for financing Britain's deficits with the USA and Europe. This was possible because Britain had a surplus with India and a huge deficit with the rest of the world, while India had a deficit with Britain and a huge surplus with the rest of the world. (pp. 80–81)

The experiences of the last 70 years tell a completely different story. When we compare the general well-being of the people of South Asia with that of the residents of other regions, the results are disturbing. Though these sovereign nations exhibit a strong commitment to improving the well-being of their respective populations, conditions have not improved as expected, whether we look at income, health, education, or governance. Overall, Sri Lanka, which shares a colonial history similar to that of India and the rest of the subcontinent, achieved nearly universal education and health care despite years of militancy and war (UNDP, 2014, p. 87). This achievement has been marred by prevalent corruption.

Hsieh and Klenow (2009) reported that if resource allocation in China and India were as efficient as it is in the United States, productivity would increase by as much as 50% in China and 60% in India. In the last half-century, resource allocation has been a considerable challenge for South Asia. Using a monetary indicator as a measure of well-being assumes that individuals or households can freely reallocate their resources among consumption, health, and education. If so, measuring the amount of resources available to individuals or households is enough to assess the maximum well-being they can attain (Martin, Béteille, Li, Mitra, & Newman, 2015, p. 45). Availability of choices would facilitate better living conditions for all residents.

GDP as a measure of progress has been under scrutiny by many and alternative measures are being developed. In India, former president Pranab Mukherjee has stated that increase in GDP is not commensurate with an increase in happiness so an alternative measure is necessary. Burchardt (2013) states that by following conventional measures of progress like GDP, much that is relevant to the health of an economy is omitted, the most important perhaps of which are household production and unpaid work. So in the example of childcare, if the boundary between the formal market and informal market (for example, parental) shifts towards the former, this would show up as an increase in GDP, even though the amount of caring activity remains unchanged. The South Asian region is experiencing the same phenomenon. A detailed note on GDP and alternative measurements has been put in Chap. 5 of this book.

4.3 Health, Hygiene and Hindrances—Towards Human Well-Being in South Asia

The poor health outcomes in South Asia can be attributed to low expenditures on health and lack of an adequate health care infrastructure, especially in the rural areas where around two-thirds of the region's population reside. A contributing factor to poor life expectancy is the comparatively low level of public investment in local, regional, and national health services as discussed in Chap. 3. Out-of-pocket household expense on health in the South Asian region is around four times more than the world average. The gap in the public allocation of funds for improving health has adversely affected the parameters used to measure health well-being.

South Asia has the world's largest number of malnourished children. Inadequate nutrition adversely affects the development of the brain and cognitive faculties. These children enter the education system with huge initial learning disadvantages, and the effects are compounded over time. Dundar, Beteille, Riboud, and Deolalikar (2014) argue for a multisectoral approach to assure good nutrition for children entering schools. The South Asian governments have introduced different programs (e.g., mid-day meal plan, etc.) to sufficiently improve health conditions for schooling. This region rates somewhat better than Sub-Saharan Africa in terms of health parameters; otherwise, its overall level of health performance ranks far behind every other subregion of the world. This ranking reflects decades of neglect on the part of central and local governments in developing health infrastructures. India's famed traditional healing systems of Ayurveda and similar types of innovative medicine have contributed relatively little to advances in public or communal health. The steps taken in India to strengthen the reach of Ayurveda, Yoga and Naturopathy, Unani, Siddha, and Homeopathy under the Ministry of AYUSH to the wider part of the country are helping broaden the healthcare system there. The last decade has witnessed a proliferation of Ayurvedic products, and the Indian government has promoted private sector investment in health, especially in supporting Yoga and Ayurveda.

In December 2014, the United Nations General Assembly recognized the importance of yoga for better well-being and hence declared June 21 as International Yoga Day. Though South Asia's expenditure on healthcare has increased steadily, the resulting modest gains have been sidelined by the high rates of population growth in almost all South Asian countries, e.g., Pakistan, Nepal, Afghanistan, and Sri Lanka— all of which rank among the lowest in the world in terms of national public sector spending on health as a percentage of GDP.

The government in India has launched many initiatives to improve health care.[7] Some of them have been previously mentioned in Chap. 3. India has been focusing on ensuring affordable healthcare for all the citizens. It has established wellness centers as part of the *Ayushman Bharat* initiative for vulnerable families. The *Poshan* campaign launched to handle malnutrition. The National Health Protection Scheme provides INR five lakh (approx. USD 7000) in health coverage to families for secondary and tertiary care. The scheme is committed to eliminating tuberculosis from India, ahead of the global target. There are nearly 850 thousand ASHA (Accredited Social Health Activist) workers working under NRHM spread across the country. These are just some of the important initiatives India has taken to assure better health well-being at a national level. In India, there are disparities in health parameters by geographical region, as well as between the poor and the rich (Mahal, 2003). Some states like Kerala are doing much better than states like Uttar Pradesh.

---

[7] See https://48months.mygov.in/themes/healthy-india/accessed on November 27, 2018.

Sri Lanka, an exceptional country in South Asia, performed extremely well on health parameters despite its internal governance problems. In 2000, the global burden of diarrhea and malnutrition—attributable to climate change—was highest in India, Bangladesh, Nepal, Bhutan, and the Maldives and is expected to remain the same until 2030 (IPCC, 2007). South Asia faces major health challenges: poor sanitation, poor maternal health, poor access to healthcare services, and the prevalence of many emerging chronic diseases. Bhutan is facing a challenging time due to the allocation of its health budget and as health technologies are improving in the world, it is lagging behind. Adhikari (2016) suggests following evidence-based resource allocation to address this issue for which the Health Technology Assessment can help immensely with in terms of health financing.

SAARC has undertaken many initiatives[8] designed to improve public responses to health hazards, diseases, and other health-related problems. Though many research institutions[9] have been established in the region, many scholars (see Peters & Yazbeck, 2003; Sadana, D'Souza, Hyder, & Chowdhury, 2004; etc.) have observed that health research has not matured in this region and that it will take time for health to become a priority. The GFHR (2001) called the research gap in developing countries the "10/90 gap," whereby a meagre 10% of health research funding is allocated to 90% of the disease burden facing the world.

Since lapses often occur when implementing programs, the whole region ofSouth Asia struggles with questions of how to implement the existing and proposed programs and how to effectively reach out to needy people. Corruption at different levels is a major hindrance in effectively reaching the masses. In Bangladesh and Nepal, government health providers were pressured to provide free medicine to people whom they knew were not ill but who were selling it to others or who wanted it for livestock (World Bank, 2015a, p. 195). In some of the states in India, scams are perpetrated by very people who are supposed to deliver state-proposed expenditures to the people. A former prime minister of India once said that in India only 10% of the expenditure reaches the people for whom it was meant (Basu, 2006, p. 216).

Although South Asia has experienced some improvements in the parameters related to health well-being, the region has not been able to keep pace with improvements in other regions of the world. Though government expenditures for health as a percentage of GDP have not increased significantly, private expenditures have increased substantially. This reflects the concern for health well-being among the general public and their improved awareness level. This is also likely caused by the lack of sufficient expenditure by respective governments. Health outcomes for Sri

---

[8]The SAARC Tuberculosis and HIV/AIDS Centre was established in 1992 in Nepal, with the goal of treating and preventing tuberculosis. This center coordinates and implements regional activities related to TB and HIV/AIDS. The health ministers of the member countries of SAARC meet periodically to review progress and to develop strategies to improve the health well-being of the residents of the region. Steps are underway to develop the Telemedicine Network Project for resource sharing within the region.

[9]Bangladesh Medical Research Council, 1972; Health Research and Epidemiology Unit, Bhutan, 1995; Indian Council for Medical Research, 1911; Pakistan Medical Research Council, 1962; Nepal Health Research Council, 1991; National Health Research Council, Sri Lanka 1996.

Lanka and the Maldives are excellent whereas those for Pakistan and Afghanistan are poor. India, which contains around three-fourths of the population of the region, has a much greater challenge to improve health indicators. Though the Maldives is the smallest country in the region and maintains some of the best health parameters, it recognizes many challenges related to the health sector that they must address in the future. Some of the major challenges[10] as identified by them are:

- Lack of skilled local health professionals at all levels of the health system due to limited training opportunities in the country as well as abroad.
- Low community participation in preventive and protective health services and underutilization of the skills of trained community based public health workers.
- Inequity in access to health services.
- Lack of appropriate laws to protect public health and the human right to health.
- Limited capacity and scope of mental health programs resulting in increasing suicides, antisocial behavior, and violence.
- Emergence of communicable diseases due to climate change and human practices.
- Increase in chronic non-communicable diseases such as cardiovascular diseases, chronic respiratory diseases, and cancers due to sedentary lifestyles, obesity, and tobacco use.

Surprisingly, many people feel that public spending on health is directed more towards people who are financially secure than to the poorest population groups. Further, that public spending is progressive at the lower levels but regressive at secondary and especially tertiary levels (Martin et al., 2015, p. 97). The World Development Report 2014 (World Bank, 2013) mentioned that in South Asia, more people have cellular phones than toilets, which exemplifies the priorities that governments have had to deal with on a basic issue like this. The WaterAid, Australia published a report titled "Out of Order—The State of the World's Toilets 2017"[11] in November 2017 which brings out some more startling facts about a very basic need, the availability of toilets. According to this report, around 2.3 billion people worldwide do not have access to a toilet. The report further mentions that around 56% of the Indian population does not have access to basic sanitation facilities. South Asia has three countries in the list of 10 worst countries on the ranking for access to basic sanitation—India, Bangladesh, and Pakistan. Conversely, Nepal, Pakistan, and India are ranked in the top 10 best countries who have reduced open defecation. As per this report Nepal has reduced open defecation during 2000–2015 by 34.8%, Pakistan by 29.9%, and India by 26.1%.

The government of India, through its flagship *Swachh Bharat Mission* (Clean India Campaign), which received USD 1.5 billion from the World Bank, has made a huge positive impact on sanitation through publicity and awareness programs and by

---

[10] Accessed from http://www.health.gov.mv/Uploads/Downloads//Informations/Informations(54).pdf on November 27, 2018.

[11] See https://www.wateraid.org/uk/sites/g/files/jkxoof211/files/Out%20of%20Order%20report%202017_0.pdf retrieved on December 24, 2017.

providing financial support for the construction of toilets. In last four years the Clean India Campaign has been able to make more than 550 thousand villages defecation free and constructed more than 10 million toilets.[12] It is projected that by the 150th birthday of Mahatma Gandhi (October 2, 2019), India will end open defecation. Examining the current progress, this goal is achievable and will possibly be achieved even earlier. In Nepal, investments in sanitation are contributing significantly to preventing anemia[13] (Coffey, Geruso, & Spears, 2018). Overall in South Asia region the inequalities in health outcomes are wide (Martin et al., 2015). It is caused due to limited access to basic care among the poor and more so for pregnant women. The slow pace of health well-being is attributable to the region's continuing high rates of fertility and increasing years of average life expectancy. Reducing fertility rate has also been one of the priorities for health policy makers. Much has to improve in the domain of public funding for health services on count of availability and quality of service. South Asia has a long way to go to substantially improve the health well-being of its people.

4.4 Education, Empowerment, and Entitlement—Towards Human Well-Being in South Asia

Education improves empowerment. Education in itself is also considered empowerment. Good education instills a sense of responsibility towards society and well-being. It infuses a sense of commitment towards the cause of nation building apart from making an individual ready to earn living. Education and empowerment expand entitlement which enhances HWB. The South Asia region has been striving hard to improve educational well-being through the policies and their effective implementation. Though all the countries of the region are prioritizing "Education for All" through their own initiatives, it is a significant challenge for most of them to achieve. The Maldives and Sri Lanka are exceptions to this as they have been able to reach more than a 90% literacy level. For the most part, the public expenditure on education in the region is abysmally low and the private sector is more interested in quick return over investment—hence quality is being significantly compromised. Yet the contribution of philanthropies and missionaries towards improving education conditions in the region is considerable. Participation of private entrepreneurs in the education sector is on the rise across South Asia, except for Bhutan, where only a few private schools (and only in some urban pockets) are available for middle-level education. Education is starting to be considered an important business opportunity, and it is becoming part of public-private partnership ventures. This trend is, however, occurring only in urban areas; ironically, about 67% of the total population of South Asia still resides in rural villages. Unlike in ancient times (3000 BC to 1000 AD)

---

[12] As available from https://transformingindia.mygov.in/performance-dashboard/#primary.

[13] As cited in World Bank (2018, p. 53).

when education was considered necessary for building character, gaining knowledge, creating learned societies, and spreading scholarship to the other parts of the world; today education is considered necessary only as preparation to earn a living in the market-driven economy. The great institutions of this region, such as Takshila (now in Pakistan) and Nalanda (now in India), which developed a strong culture of learning, knowledge, and wisdom, have lost their relevance in modern times. Efforts are underway to revive Nalanda as world class university.

In order to improve education well-being, the major challenge is to improve the quality of education for which improving the quality of teachers is perhaps the most significant way. The improvement in the quality of teachers shall lead to improve learning outcomes, and its benefits are expected to translate into national economic gains (Dundar et al., 2014). Institutions of higher learning are available and affordable, albeit the quality is highly varied. Bhutan and Bangladesh were among the first 20 countries to sign and ratify the UN Convention on the Rights of the Child under the Education for All Summit in 1990 (Bajaj & Kidwai, 2016). Now all the eight countries of the region are signatories to the convention and are trying to improve the educational standards discussed in Chap. 3.

Bangladesh has made remarkable gains in ensuring access to education in the past two decades. As of 2015, the country's net enrolment rate at the primary school level is above 90%, and secondary school level is around 62%. With nearly 6.4 million girls in secondary school in 2015, Bangladesh is among the few countries to achieve gender parity in school enrolment, and has more girls than boys in secondary schools.[14]

ILO reports[15] that there are around 30 million children employed in the work force which includes 17 million child laborers and it is estimated that around 50 million children are out of school across South Asia. Child labor conditions have been worsening in the region. In these challenging times Kailash Satyarthi (Box 4.1) has fought for children's rights and his initiatives aimed towards protecting child rights and improving the living conditions of children have gained momentum. His services to humanity have been globally recognized.

Box 4.1
Brief Profile of Kailash Satyarthi
Poverty often deprives children from the chance to attend school and instead forces them to work and earn for the family. More than 10% of children across the world have been found to be involved in child labor. South Asia has the largest number of children working among any region. Estimations by the ILO state that 16.7 million (5–17 years old) children are working as child laborers in South Asia. There are around 5.8 million children in India, 5 million

---

[14]See https://www.worldbank.org/en/region/sar/overview#3 as updated on Jul 16, 2018.
[15]See   https://www.ilo.org/newdelhi/areasofwork/child-labour/WCMS_300805/lang--en/index.htm. All children employed do not fall under the category of child labor. The ILO defines child labor as work that deprives children of their childhood, their potential and their dignity, and that is harmful to physical and mental development.

in Bangladesh, 3.4 million in Pakistan, and 2 million in Nepal who are all involved in child labor.[16] The conditions of child labor in Nepal, Bangladesh, and Pakistan are worse than other nations when the participation of children in total labor force is taken into consideration. Discovering these facts and prompted by conscience, Kailash Satyarthi took a vow to save children from this menace and instead put them in school.

Kailash Satyarthi is a child rights activist and a Nobel Prize winner for his work fighting against the oppression of children and for the right to education for all. He has been a guiding light in the global movement against child slavery and exploitation and has relentlessly worked to free thousands of children exploited by businessmen, landowners, and others since 1980. As an activist, he founded the 'Bachpan Bachao Andolan' (BBA) or Save the Childhood Movement—against the child labor widely practiced all across the world, but more particularly in India.[17] Satyarthi gave up his lucrative job as an engineer and dedicated his life to work to ensuring human well-being.

In 1988, he led the global march against child labor—an 80,000 km-long march across 103 countries—to raise awareness against modern child slavery. It became one of the largest social movements on behalf of exploited children. The BBA liberated children who had been forced into servitude and slavery and also established ashrams for them to re-acclimate and start their education. Satyarthi urged international cooperation which led to the formation of South Asian Coalition on Child Servitude (SACCS) in 1989 which collaborated with various unions and NGOs in India, Bangladesh, Nepal, and Sri Lanka[18] for liberating child labors in South Asia. SACCS has been able to liberate more than 40,000 children to date.

Kailash Satyarthi launched RugMark (GoodWeave), which certifies that carpets are not woven by children.[19] RugMark has created awareness among customers and positively impacts buying decisions. Satyarthi was the co-founder of the Global Campaign for Education and became the founding member of the UNESCO High-Level Group on Education for All in 2001. He has been serving on various committees and boards including the Centre for Victims of Torture in US and the International Labor Rights Fund.[20]

In 2014, he was awarded the Nobel Peace Prize for his sustained efforts to end child labor, human trafficking, exploitation, and improving human

---

[16]See   https://www.ilo.org/newdelhi/areasofwork/child-labour/WCMS_300805/lang--en/index. htm.

[17]See   https://timesofindia.indiatimes.com/city/chandigarh/satyarthi-to-deliver-talk-in-pu-on-oct-12/articleshow/60988413.cms.

[18]See   https://www.aljazeera.com/news/asia/2014/10/profile-kailash-satyarthi-2014101012382235808.html.

[19]See https://goodweave.org/.

[20]See https://www.outlookindia.com/magazine/story/who-will-save-the-children/292301.

well-being by promoting education for all.[21] His persistent efforts received international support when child protection and welfare related clauses were included in the Sustainable Development Goals of the United Nations in 2015.[22] He launched Bharat Yatra to spread awareness about child rape and trafficking, which covered 12,000 km across 22 Indian states and union territories. More than 1200 thousand marchers participated in the campaign and led to the passage of the Criminal Law (Amendment) Bill in 2018 which paved the way for time-bound trials and stringent punishments for the rapists of minor girls.[23]

He also initiated the global movement for an international law against digital forms of child sexual abuse and exploitation around the world. In 2018, the Indian government banned 857 pornographic websites following his demands towards ending child pornography and sexual abuse.[24] He was the subject of an award-winning documentary named "The Price of Free" that showed his daring rescue operations and spread awareness about child abuse.[25] He has been the recipient of numerous awards and honors such as the Santokhba Humanitarian Award (2018), Harvard University's "Humanitarian of the Year" award (2015), Defenders of Democracy Award (2009), etc. Satyarthi continues to demonstrate courage amid death threats and strives to ensure human well-being by relentlessly campaigning for an exploitation-free world for children. He has been able to sensitize society to the ill effects of child labor and to inspire many countrymen to contribute towards human well-being through their own initiatives.

His crusade has impacted lives of children in India immensely and his contribution towards developing facilitating legal framework and its implementation shall certainly guide future policies.

The conditions of higher education are not satisfactory in South Asia as compared to the standards of other regions. The quality of teachers is an issue that plagues this region as a whole. This concern has added to the slow and/or poor improvement in education-related indicators. A Goldman Sachs report found that India scored poorly relative to BRICS (Brazil, Russia, India, China, and South Africa) and scored below

---

[21] See   http://www.firstpost.com/india/why-indias-kailash-satyarthi-won-the-2014-nobel-peace-prize-all-you-need-to-know-1751057.html.

[22] See   http://in.one.un.org/page/un-public-lecture-on-sustainable-development-begins-with-education/.

[23] See   https://www.sentinelassam.com/news/new-bill-will-end-india-as-transit-point-for-trafficking-of-girls-says-nobel-laureate-kailash-satyarthi/.

[24] See   https://www.indiawest.com/news/india/satyarthi-meets-pope-to-discuss-international-law-against-online-child/article_8229c9fc-e9dc-11e8-b2e5-7b36218a2c6e.html.

[25] See   https://indiacurrents.com/giving-tuesday-kailash-satyarthi-award-winning-youtube-documentary-released/.

the average relative to emerging economies in terms of school quality. Additionally, India's growth and productivity were negatively affected by low educational standards across the board (O'Neill & Poddar, 2008). As mentioned previously, though there are political commitments toward education for all, they have not effectively reached the masses. The relationship between teachers and politicians has negatively influenced teacher quality and accountability in government schools in India (Beteille, 2009). Political interference in the functioning of schools and involvement of teachers in political activities has affected the quality of inputs and delivery. Militancy also hinders educational reform in some parts of South Asia. In Nepal, the civil conflict due to recent Maoist insurgency has adversely affected education for girls, but overall it has not significantly reduced the number of years of education for either boys or girls (Valente, 2011). Many households do not send their children to schools, especially their daughters, in Afghanistan and Pakistan.

In Pakistan, many girls who wish to attend school must deal with two types of social boundaries: caste boundaries and gender boundaries. Low-caste girls may face discrimination if they attend a school dominated by high castes, and all girls are subject to *purdah*, a form of female seclusion that restricts women's mobility and social interactions. These social constraints limit educational opportunities available to girls (World Bank, 2015b: 52). On one side the world is targeting on improvement of quality of education and equity, this region still has not achieved education for all targets.

The World Bank (2011) reported that, although overall enrolment has improved, many fewer girls—and members of other disadvantaged groups—than boys are enrolled in primary and secondary schools in many sub-Saharan countries and some parts of South Asia. In Bangladesh, India, Nepal, and Sri Lanka, religion explains part of the inequality in access to primary education. In India, caste explains this more so than religion (Martin et al., 2015, p. 111) because caste dominates religion regarding inequality in access to primary education. Though schooling in Nepal is improving, the improvement has not yet sufficiently addressed the diversities of caste, language, gender, class, and recently, political affiliation. Due to frequent changes in the political system over the past 70 years, the country does not have a consistent priority and policy in terms of education. Historically, the monarchy in Nepal considered education the prerogative of the ruling elite and made no attempts to extend schooling to all citizens (Bajaj & Kidwai, 2016). The idea that all human beings, irrespective of caste, creed, color, or religion, are equal should be instilled in the minds of all children. In this context, the roles and responsibilities of parents and teachers are crucial.

Many of the region's people, especially the young people, are unemployed; some migrate to other parts of the world in search of improved economic opportunities. The brain drain phenomenon is visibly prevalent across South Asia. Dependency on foreign remittance is widespread throughout the region as well. These remittances are not sustainable and the conditions of poor living conditions are prevalent across. Political instability work as a disincentive for different governments of the region to provide income security for the region's historically most vulnerable populations, e.g., widows and their children; the aged; unemployed workers; persons belonging to socially disadvantaged groups; and persons with chronic illnesses or permanent disabilities that prevent them from working. The government expects families, neighbors, local communities, and religious organizations to provide for the basic material needs of these persons—albeit many remain outside the care of even these informal systems of social welfare. Poverty is widespread and highly visible in most of the countries of South Asia, as are begging and the disfigurement of children to increase their value as beggars.

Overall, poverty in Bangladesh, the country with the highest levels in South Asia, is seemingly the single largest factor explaining why outcomes fail to match policy goals concerning the right to (primary) education in the country (Bajaj & Kidwai, 2016). Sub-Saharan Africa has the greatest inequality in health whereas South Asia has the greatest inequality in education (UNDP, 2013, p. 14). Education that leads towards empowering citizens and making them capable to prove their entitlements through knowledge, skills and abilities needs to be provided to the youth of the region. Overdependence on the state for the creation of job opportunities has affected the expectation level of youth. The World Bank Education Strategy 2020[26] which targets access, equity, quality, and governance, will be a reality only when employment opportunities for students improve. Apart from improving employment opportunities vocational education and skill development programs shall help empower youth to take up jobs. Most of the countries of the region are putting up systems to improve infrastructural conditions of skill development.

It is expected that India will have highest youth working population in the coming two decades. Taking that into consideration, if the educational standards are not immediately improved, the future is bleak for India. The governments of all the countries of the region must firmly commit to improving the quality of education, more so in countries like India, Pakistan, and Bangladesh which constitute more than 95% of the regional population. These steps shall help improve entitlements resulting in enhancing human well-being.

4.5 Politics, Policy, and Governance—Towards Human Well-Being in South Asia

The government—through laws and regulations—puts a system in place to develop, design, and deliver effective policies for the welfare of its citizens, vis-à-vis., state. Elected governments face greater challenges as compared to monarchs or dictators because citizens elect them, hence they need to be responsive to cater to the needs of the people. Today, more and more nations are becoming democracies, by compulsion or by choice. In democratic systems it is the choice of people as to what kind of government they want. Availability of choice to the people and diligent use of that choice by the people make democratic system strong and responsible. It is in this

---

[26] Accessed from http://siteresources.worldbank.org/EDUCATION/Resources/ESSU/463292-1306181142935/WB_ES_ExectiveSummary_FINAL.pdf.

Table 4.2 A changing world: rise in number of electoral democracies

Region	1990	2000	2014
Countries under electoral democracies	76	120	125
Developing countries under democracies	49	89	95
East Asia and Pacific	10	16	18
Europe and Central Asia	3	18	19
Latin America and the Caribbean	28	29	29
Middle East and North Africa	1	1	2
South Asia	3	4	7
Sub-Saharan Africa	4	21	20

Source Freedom House (Lateef, 2016, p. 29)

context that one can say that progression from compulsion to choice ideally lead towards building developed societies. It is also applied in economic theories where in fair market system, availability of choices to a customer lead to converting sellers' market into buyers' market.

The governments have to manage and allocate resources to draw effective policy for the state and its people leading towards assurance of HWB. The implementation and delivery of these policies become extremely crucial (especially in the South Asian region) where rules, laws, regulations, etc., have to facilitate efficient execution of the policies. The background paper to the World Development Report 2017 as written by Lateef (2016) provides interesting facts and analysis advocating for the need for governance measures in order to more effectively reach out to intended populations in a free environment where government is held highly accountable and adherence to law is basic. Here political governance becomes the key. Lateef (2016, p. 29), through the data of change in electoral democracies (Table 4.2), argues that the developing world has undergone more integration and progressed relatively faster economically. The whole world is moving towards organized societies built through democratic practices. Between 1990 and 2014 the number of electoral democracies has risen from 76 to 125. South Asia has a very diverse story to share with the world. The economic progress in some cases is much better than others, in some cases governance and political stability is much better but not economic growth. Some nations are behind in terms of ensuring and maintaining the basic tenets of democracy, despite the fact that most of these countries have adopted democracy as the form of governance (Jamil, Askvik, & Dhakal, 2013).

In Chap. 3, the status of all South Asian countries in governance as per World Governance Indicators was discussed by looking at each variable of the index. Poor governance and corruption undermine good performance in economic growth and steadiness in other indicators. The primary cause of poor governance in South Asia is due to poor educational standards and lack of awareness of rights and entitlements among the masses. Politicians often exploit the electorates by making false promises and practicing dishonest measures such as misinformation and manipu-lation. Political instability in most of these countries has negatively affected policy implementation and social progress. *The Himalayan Times*, in its November 24, 2017 edition said: "In Nepal, bureaucracy or public sectors have suffered most from the rampant corruption. In fiscal year 2015–16, the Commission for the Investigation of Abuse of Authority (CIAA), Nepal received a total of 15,126 cases of corruption. Among these cases, most came from the department of education, local develop-ment, and health."[27] There is a collective failure of execution machinery in Nepal which is causing a large gap between policy and performance. Trends are similar across the region. Governance in education and health is most important as it is a base of social infrastructure and concerns future of any country, and unfortunately it is compromised in the region.

The word "politics" has a different connotation in most of South Asia compared to the rest of the world, and often unfavorably viewed. The nations of South Asia have many different forms of government—democratic, socialist, military, and monar-chical. Military rule, monarchy, and a centralized autocratic political system are accepted within the framework of democracy in the region (Nepali, 2009, p. 5). Many schemes and programs though intended to benefit the common citizens, do not reach to the masses. This is also due to corrupt bureaucrats and politicians. Favoritism and lawlessness run rampant. According to the World Justice Project,[28] Pakistan and Afghanistan are among the bottom 10 countries wherein people are most likely to break the law to increase their own comfort and by their choice—rather than what is expected by law. As reported in the World Development Report 2017, rule of law is highly correlated with high income countries, as the Rule of Law Index shows much higher values for OECD countries as compared to the countries in Sub-Saharan Africa and South Asia (World Bank, 2017, p. 96). However, Bhutan has been very successful in maintaining rule of law even though it falls in the low-income category. This is partly because Bhutan's concern has not been on increasing GDP, rather it has focused on happiness of people, vis-à-vis., HWB (also see Shrotryia, 2017). Bhutan's journey of GNH has been briefly described in Annexure.

The prevalence of crime, violence, terrorism, and militarization consumes signif-icant resources which includes precious human resource and capital. Huge amount of useful political energy is wasted in dealing with these issues which ultimately negatively affect social indicators. The countries which spend more on public ser-vices tend to reduce insurgent violence, as data from India and Afghanistan proves (Beath, Christia, & Enikolopov, 2012; Khanna & Zimmermann, 2015). However, it is important to mention that in the case of Afghanistan, the reduction in violence was short-lived and limited in areas with initially low levels of violence (World Bank, 2017, p. 120). It is also believed that naxalism, violence, and terrorism are signs of poor governance, hence if governance is improved and trust and confidence is built, destructive activism would be significantly reduced.

---

[27] See 'Governance in Nepal' in https://thehimalayantimes.com/opinion/good-governance-new-hopes retrieved on August 28, 2018.

[28] See https://worldjusticeproject.org/.

Decentralization plays a major role in developing better governance systems. Through effective local governance mechanisms, democratic practices can be strengthened from the ground level upwards. India, Bhutan, and Sri Lanka all have local active governance. In Bhutan, villages and blocks are politically represented, and their participation in decision making is transparent and vibrant. Sri Lanka through its elected provincial councils engages with the people at the ground level. Revival of the *Panchayat* system in India through 73rd constitutional amendment in 1992 resulted in widespread local participation in government. In the *Panchayat* system, one-third of the total political seats are reserved for women. This system provides a large political platform for women, thereby impacting the lives of all women in the region by empowering them to express their views in the development of their communities. Despite initiatives in the region to decentralize, South Asia continues to encounter challenges such as inadequate resources, political interventions, inconsistent practices, and a low level of stakeholder engagement.

The Right to Information (RTI) and Right to Education (RTE) Act's in India were pushed through by public movements which stemmed from the *Panchayats* system. These acts have helped poor and vulnerable citizens demand better services and education for their children, thus improving living conditions within slums (World Bank, 2017, p. 20). The RTI Act was the result of more than a decade of efforts by rural activists who brought together disparate stakeholders ultimately culminating into the historic legislation (ibid., p. 241). Proactive and constructive activism at local levels of governance also helps build the credibility of individual leaders to prepare them for assuming larger roles. These individual leaders become change makers at policy and implementation level in national politics for the cause of HWB. This is true in case of Joko Widodo of Indonesia as well as Narendra Modi of India, who have both held offices at local (or provincial) levels by winning the trust of people at the ground level, and later occupied offices at the national level. "Decentralized democracies allow opposition political parties to gain support in specific localities or regions and eventually to challenge the dominant national party. In India, the Bharatiya Janata Party, which carried Modi into the national government, gained strength over time by winning several elections at the state level" (Rudolph & Rudolph, 2001).[29]

Till 2014, India was led by an economist prime minister, Man Mohan Singh from Indian National Congress. India changed leadership in 2014. The major impetus of this change was the alleged corruption and crony capitalism charges leveled against the previous administration. The government completed its term successfully in 2019. In the general elections held in 2019, people voted for the same political party showing their trust and loyalty to the government led by Narendra Modi. The most recent government administration has implemented many transformative changes during its tenure. Under general protests over prevalent frequent rapes, the government enacted a law giving the death penalty to convicted rapists. In order to empower women in the villages, provisions were made to make mandatory for reservation of seats for

---

[29] As cited in World Bank (2017, p. 218).

women in village panchayats[30] for their participation in decision making at local government level. Child labor regulations have improved working conditions. In order to smoothen the process of governance, the present government repealed many irrelevant acts which had become obsolete and were causing bureaucratic inconvenience. Demonetization and implementation of the Goods and Services Tax by the Indian government is claimed to have resulted in positive economic growth, though it also resulted in protests among the masses (especially demonetization) when it was introduced. Demonetization and the Goods and Services Tax had helped encourage formalizing of informal sector. It has been possible to push the use of technology for financial transactions resulting in significant reduction in cash transactions. Primarily demonetization has been able to unearth a myriad of fake firms and has been able to curb corruption to great extent. As reported[31] on May 2018, more than 730 hundred companies that were deregistered, deposited more than INR 24,000 crore (approx. USD 5.1 billion) in bank accounts post-demonetization, and the ministry of corporate affairs has removed the names of around 226 hundred thousand companies.

Governance has been a severe problem in the region as a whole but things have begun to change in some of the countries of the region. The new government in Nepal is completing two years (2017 election); the governments in Afghanistan, Bhutan, The Maldives, and Pakistan are yet to complete a year (2018 election); people in Bangladesh and India have elected their governments in 2019 only. Politics in all these countries has defined the policy paradigm and so is a priority for providing good governance. It has been difficult for many to effectively connect to the masses. It has also been hard for them to counter corruption, increase accountability, and implement a policy of transparency. Things have begun to improve with the use of technology assuring efficiency and timely resolve of problems. An active network of NGOs is able to raise voice and concern which is adding strength to the future course of action. Until governance is improved, even good parameters in terms of education and health will not be successful.

4.6 Conclusion

While addressing the nation on the national day of Bhutan, the king of Bhutan gave an honest and confessional statement: "We Bhutanese are good at writing plans, speaking well, and expounding ideas. But implementation falls short of commitments. There is a gap between commitments made and output delivered. We are not able to deliver results of expected quality in a timely manner" (GNHC, 2017, p. 13). The same sentiment can be applied to most South Asian countries. More efficient

---

[30] It was observed that women participation in general at local governance level (village panchayat) was negligible. Hence mandatory provision for women participation have been made.

[31] *The Times of India* published on June 4, 2018, also available at: https://timesofindia. indiatimes.com/business/india-business/73000-deregistered-cos-deposited-rs-24000-crore-post-demonetisation-govt-data/articleshow/64437555.cms?utm_source=contentofinterest&utm_medium=text&utm_campaign=cppst.

delivery systems and effective execution of policy and programs are the keys which need serious attention and commitment. It is evident that much needs to be done to improve the well-being of the people of South Asia (also see Shrotryia, 2017). Governments in the region have not been able to implement and monitor projects deigned to improve living conditions of their citizens successfully. The countries must increase public spending on health and education in order to see a long-term improvement. Improving health and education parameters, thereby empowering the population economically, will benefit everyone. The people of these countries will develop a sense of pride in their respective nationalities from increased positive indicators, which should improve their overall life satisfaction.

In this region, social and local identities are stronger than national identities. India is a Hindu majority secular state and, though clashes have occurred between Muslims and Hindus, a harmonious coexistence is also evident in many areas of the country. Other parts of the region also have minority-majority conflicts, for example, the Tamil and Sinhalese in Sri Lanka and Shia-Sunni conflict in Pakistan, including the threat from the Balochs.[32] As mentioned earlier, diversity is embedded in the basic fabric of the region. Among the eight countries of South Asia, India is the most diverse in terms of language, ethnicity, religion, caste, and tribe. The education, health, and economic well-being of disadvantaged groups in India have posed a significant challenge to the state in terms of devising and implementing programs to improve their well-being. The Constitution of India includes provisions to safeguard the interests of people belonging to educationally and socially disadvantaged groups because of their caste. They have been formally grouped in three categories: Scheduled Castes (SCs), Schedule Tribes (STs), and Other Backward Class (OBCs). Together, they comprise more than 50% of the population. These groups have a low level of general well-being because they live under poor educational, health, and economic conditions. For this reason, successive governments have advocated and implemented a job reservation policy (a proxy for affirmative action) for these groups of people. This has resulted in providing them with better employment opportunities and in improving their well-being. The country as a whole witnessed a significant transformation well-being because today members of these groups hold key positions in government as well as in private institutions. Dirks (2001, p. 3) rightly stated that "when thinking of India, it is hard not to think of caste. ...caste has become a central symbol for India."

Muni (1979) identified several factors that obstructed the development of regionalism in South Asia which were colonial legacies, problems of national integration, nation building, unequal economic development and regime stability, power disparities in the region superimposed by an artificial balance between India and Pakistan, and the role of external powers. Ironically, South Asia has not yet been able to rise above these issues, which has a negative effect on the general well-being of people.

There are two India's: One is a new, vibrant, globally competitive India, based on the knowledge industries—software, the internet, information technology-enabled services, generic pharmaceuticals, and entertainment. It is professionally run. The

---

[32]Balochistan is one of the four states (provinces) in Pakistan. The residents of this province are referred as Balochs.

second is the old India of the family houses, which is still floundering. This segment of India has not acquired the skills needed to succeed in the global economy (Das, 2002, p. 135). The first India is still small compared to the second India.

South Asia is geographically, culturally, and religiously diverse. This diversity, sometimes considered strength, has also been a source of political conflict both past and present. There is an inverse relationship between the number of languages spoken in a particular region and the well-being of the people residing in that region (Sreekumar, 2014). Yazbeck and Peters (2003) consider South Asia as a region of contrasts when it comes to size of the countries and different indicators related to health. The region continues to struggle with military conflicts that originate both within and outside the region. These conflicts continuously threaten to disrupt the peace throughout the region and the world as a whole. SAARC, which has articulated strategies for improving the well-being of the people of the region, has a challenging role in the years to come.

Broadly this chapter facilitated a discussion on well-being outcomes (income, health, education, and governance), policy initiatives as taken up by respective governments, and outcomes as detailed in Chaps. 2 and 3. Different reports and research publications which were found to be related to human well-being and input-output items have been cited. Overall the picture of South Asia as emerges through the analysis of these items is discussed in the following concluding chapter.

Annexure: Brief on Bhutan's Journey Through Gross National Happiness Path

The kingdom of Bhutan (as it is officially called) has spearheaded the movement to include happiness in policy agenda and to prioritize it over GDP. Bhutan is a small nation of less than one million people whose government strongly believes in the happiness and general well-being of its citizens. In 1972, the Bhutanese king spoke about the importance of gross national happiness (GNH) at a United Nations gathering in Geneva. Ever since, GNH has become the foundation of socioeconomic theory in Bhutan and has guided public policy. Bhutan released a document in 1999 called the Bhutan 2020 Document[33] which provided the direction for future planning and policy execution. The document provided a normative architecture reflecting Bhutan's traditional thinking towards the maximization of GNH (Fig. 4.2).

Almost all of Bhutan's planning documents underscore the fact that GNH is the top priority of the government. Environment protection and sustainable development is recognized as one of the main objectives of government planning which is identified as an important component to maximize GNH. Maintaining forest coverage for the cause of dealing with climate change and handling carbon emission environmentally has been one of the priorities of the government. Bhutan achieved 72.5%

---

[33] See Bhutan Planning Commission (1999).

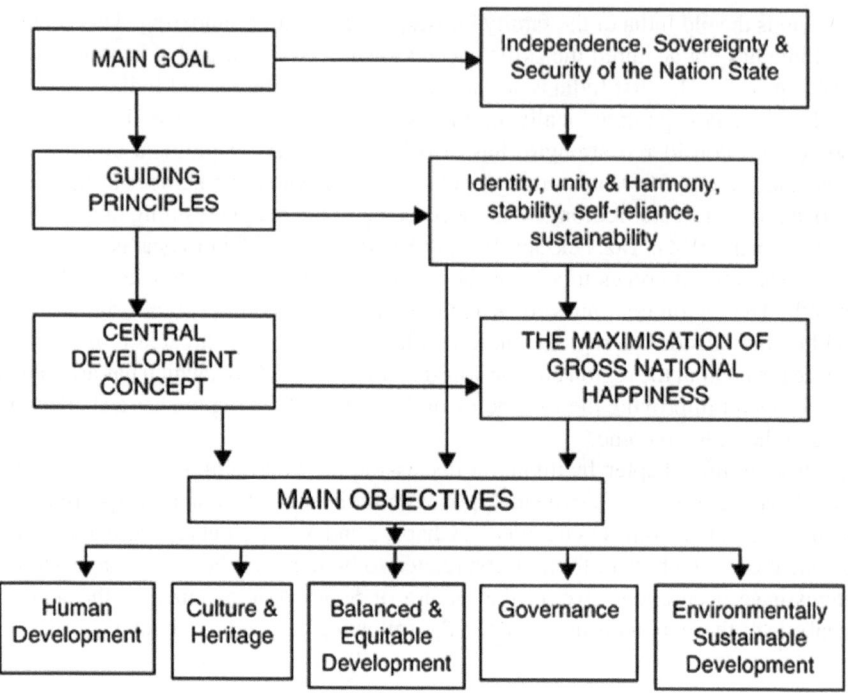

Fig. 4.2 Normative architecture for future change and development

forest coverage (United Nations, 2001) because the National Assembly (the highest legislative body in Bhutan) mandated that the country should indefinitely maintain at least 60% of its land area under forest cover (Planning Commission, 2002). A fact sheet published by the Bhutanese government in 2006 showed that a large percentage of its citizens reported a happy life status. Many of the parameters used in the survey indicated favorable conditions: access to primary health care was greater than 90%; access to safe drinking water in rural areas was about 65%; more than 90% of the children were immunized; life expectancy at birth had increased to 66 years (Planning Commission Secretariat, 2000). Bhutan was the first South Asian country to be recognized as a Normal Iodine Nutrition Country (RGOB, 2005, p. 29) and was also identified as a Millennium Development Goals fast-track country based on governance qualifications (United Nations Millennium Project, 2005, p. 234). Bhutan has been one of the most successful countries in South Asia in terms of development and the delivery of social welfare (Rutland, 1999). It has enjoyed a strong growth record over the last decade due to sound macroeconomic management, good governance, and the rapid development of hydroelectric power resources (International Monetary Fund, 2004). The philosophy of GNH is based on the quality of life (QOL) of the people, as the Planning Commission (2000, p. 20) states: "The pursuit of GNH calls for a multi-dimensional approach to development that seeks to maintain harmony and balance between economic forces, environmental preservation, cultural and spiritual values and good governance". The premise of QOL is derived from the theory that, once a person's basic human needs are fulfilled, the individual experiences positive subjective well-being (SWB). A better QOL improves the satisfaction level of people, vis-à-vis their happiness.

Rural-urban differences in QOL indicators in eastern Bhutan between 2001 and 2005 (Shrotryia, 2009) indicate that the developmental pace of physical infrastructure was faster in rural areas than urban; however, the satisfaction level did not rise correspondingly. Bhutan can attest to the fact that despite multiple constraints (of resources) and pressures (from outside world to operate in free market system), it can sustain its developmental process. The philosophy of GNH has inspired the citizens of this kingdom to maintain peace, tranquility, and sovereignty (Shrotryia, 2006). Bhutan adopted its written constitution on July 18, 2008. "The constitution became the legal framework for a democratic political system, which aimed *to secure the blessings of liberty, to ensure justice and tranquility and to enhance the unity, happiness and well-being of the people for all time*" (Phuntsho, 2013, p. 572). Article 9 (2)[34] of the constitution further states that, "the State shall strive to promote those conditions that will enable the pursuit of GNH."

Government planners concentrated on measures that would result in the happiness of people rather than just in economic growth. This mindset led to policies focused on better QOL for the people, thereby creating a happy society. As creating a happy society became a national priority in Bhutan, all ministries and departments involved in developing public policies worked with decision makers and implementing agencies to initiate and execute the policies and programs that would result in increased GNH. In order to further operationalize GHN; many workshops, seminars, and conferences were organized. These helped clarify GNH and resolved issues that were crucial to its practical application. Several international conferences and workshops were held during the first decade of the 21st century to discuss how to operationalize and measure GNH.

In 2008, the Planning Commission in Bhutan became the GNH Commission. It is headed by Bhutan's prime minister, who is assisted by both bureaucrats and policymakers. The GNH Commission tasked the Center for Bhutan Studies with developing a measuring instrument in order to gauge GNH (which later became the Center for Bhutan Studies and GNH Research, and has been declared an official institute for GNH in Bhutan). The Center published a short guide to the GNH Index and developed its first nationwide index (comprehensive GNH Index) in 2010 which measured the satisfaction level (impact of public policies on well-being of citizens) of people related to different aspects of QOL (based on nine domains, each having equal weight). The major objectives[35] for preparation of the GNH Index are identified as:

---

[34] The constitution of Bhutan was accessed from http://www.nationalcouncil.bt/assets/uploads/docs/acts/2017/Constitution_of_Bhutan_2008.pdf.

[35] See Ura, Alkire, Zangmo, and Wangdi (2015, p. 32).

- Setting an alternative framework of development.
- Providing indicators to sectors to guide development.
- Allocating resources in accordance with targets.
- Measuring people's happiness and well-being.
- Measuring progress over time.
- Comparing progress across the country.

Keeping these objectives in mind, the index was developed based on the Alkire-Foster method[36] focusing on nine domains based on normative as well as statistical data. The index uses two kinds of thresholds: sufficiency threshold and happiness threshold, and measures all of nine domains through 33 indicators (which are assigned different weights), and 102 sub-indicators (questions).

> The objectives of Bhutan and Buddhist understandings of happiness are much broader than what is referred to as 'happiness' in Western literature. Under the title of happiness in GNH comes a range of domains of human well-being. Some of these are traditional areas of social concern such as living standards, health, and education. Some are less traditional, such as time use, psychological wellbeing, culture, community vitality, and environmental diversity.[37]

The philosophy of GNH is translated into four core pillars: incorporating equitable and balanced socioeconomic development; preserving and promoting cultural and spiritual heritage; conserving the environment; and maintaining good governance in every aspect of government. Table 4.3, shows four pillars, nine domains, and 16 key result areas used to evaluate the outcome of Bhutan's public policies to improve happiness or HWB.

In 2015, five years after the first publication of the GNH index, Bhutan conducted a survey to measure the GNH of its citizens and to analyze the changes that have taken place in the subjective well-being of the residents during 2010–2015. The survey found that on a scale of zero to one, the happiness of the Bhutanese people increased from 0.743 in 2010 to 0.756 in 2015, an increase of 1.8%.[38] This is proof that, in general, quality of life is improving in Bhutan. However, the survey reports that government performance is decreasing (Fig. 4.3). Changes in the contribution of each domain to GNH index have been depicted in Fig. 4.5 and the major changes that have occurred over time as reflected in the GNH Index have been summarized in Table 4.4 however the summarized version[39] of the 2015 survey shows us the following trends:

- 91.2% of people reported experiencing happiness.

---

[36] See http://www.grossnationalhappiness.com/docs/GNH/PDFs/Sabina_Alkire_method.pdf.
[37] See http://www.grossnationalhappiness.com/docs/GNH/PDFs/Sabina_Alkire_method.pdf.
[38] See CBS and GNHR (2016, p. 2).
[39] Ibid.

Table 4.3 Gross national happiness framework

Four pillars			
Pillar one	Pillar two	Pillar three	Pillar four
Sustainable and equitable socioeconomic development	Preservation and promotion of culture	Conservation of the environment	Good governance

Nine domains			
1. Living standards	4. Cultural diversity and resilience	8. Ecological diversity	9. Good governance
2. Education	5. Community vitality		
3. Health	6. Time use		
	7. Psychological well-being		

Sixteen key result areas			
1. Sustained economic growth	5. Strengthened Bhutanese identity, social cohesion, and harmony	7. Carbon neutral/green and climate resilient development	11. Public service delivery
2. Poverty reduced and MDG Plus achieved	6. Indigenous wisdom, arts, and crafts promoted for sustainable livelihood	8. Sustainable utilization and management of natural resources	12. Democracy and governance strengthened
3. Food secured and sustained		9. Water security	13. Gender friendly environment for women's participation
4. Full employment		10. Improved disaster resilience and management mainstreamed	14. Corruption reduced
			15. Safe society
			16. Needs of vulnerable groups addressed

- 43.4% of people said that they are deeply happy.
- People are getting healthier and their living standards have improved.
- Educated people are happier compared to uneducated.
- Single and married people are happier than widowed, divorced, or separated individuals.
- People living in urban areas are happier than those living in rural areas.
- Farmers are less happy than people employed in other professions.
- Men are happier than women.

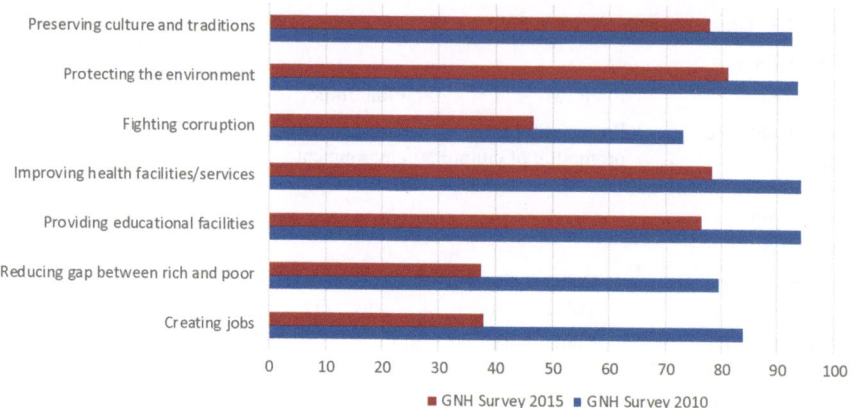

Fig. 4.3 Perception on government's performance

- Government services need to be improved as the public perception of government services has drastically gone down.
- More needs to be done to strengthen culture and traditions.
- People feel less responsible for conserving the environment.

Bhutan has concentrated its energy and resources on developing decentralized system of governance assuring wide participation. Bhutan recognizes decentralization and participation as essential elements of GNH. The number of private medical clinics is on the rise because many government doctors prefer to operate private clinics. These clinics are primarily located in urban areas. Because these clinics provide more choices to the people who can afford them, many people also feel that they contribute to a class-based society. Royal University of Bhutan was established in 2003 through a Royal Charter. Previously, the citizens of Bhutan depended on the Indian educational system because the only college in Bhutan was an affiliate of the University of Delhi, India. The Charter declared that the purpose of the university was to disseminate knowledge for the economic and cultural development of Bhutan and to promote well-being of its people.

The number of college graduates is increasing in Bhutan, which is slowly causing a rise in unemployment as opportunities are now increasing in the same way. Bhutan is developing its own information and communications technology systems; office systems are computerized and much of the official communication is performed via the Internet. With the use of ICT, Bhutan's exposure to the rest of the world has improved a lot. With the election of a democratic government, transparency and accountability of the bureaucracy have improved, and there is better communication between the citizens and their leaders. The media have become more proactive regarding issues of concern of the masses. Capital investment in infrastructure projects has increased, which has resulted in better roads and the rapid development of townships. The economy still suffers from a balance-of-payment problem caused by excess of imports

Table 4.4 GNH index 2010–2015—comparison across key indicators

Key items	GNH Index	
	2010 (N = 6476)	2015 (N = 7153)
	Figures in percent	
Deeply and extensively happy	40.9	43.4
Unhappy	10.4	8.8
Positive emotions—calmness, compassion, forgiveness, contentment, and generosity	59	51
Negative emotions—anger, fear, worry, selfishness, and jealousy	35	45
Literacy for 15–20 age group	89	95
Consider themselves 'very' spiritual	50.4	44.5
Number of people with long-term disability	13.03	15.5
Consider *Driglam Namzha* (Driglam Namzha is Bhutanese Code of Conduct and Etiquette standards) very important	93.1	92.2
Government's performance in creating jobs	83.77	37.87
Government's performance in reducing gap between rich and poor	79.46	37.42
Government's performance in protecting the environment	93.61	81.18
Trusting either most or some of their neighbors	85.3	61.6
Access to adequate drinking water	77.7	80.6
Access to electricity	72.1	96.5
Domain contribution		
Psychological well-being	11.16	10.48
Health	12.88	13.10
Time use	10.28	10.57
Education	9.60	9.78
Cultural diversity	11.05	11.01
Good governance	10.32	10.18
Community vitality	12.40	11.56
Ecological diversity	12.05	12.41
Living standard	10.26	10.91

Source Compiled from GNH 2015 survey report document

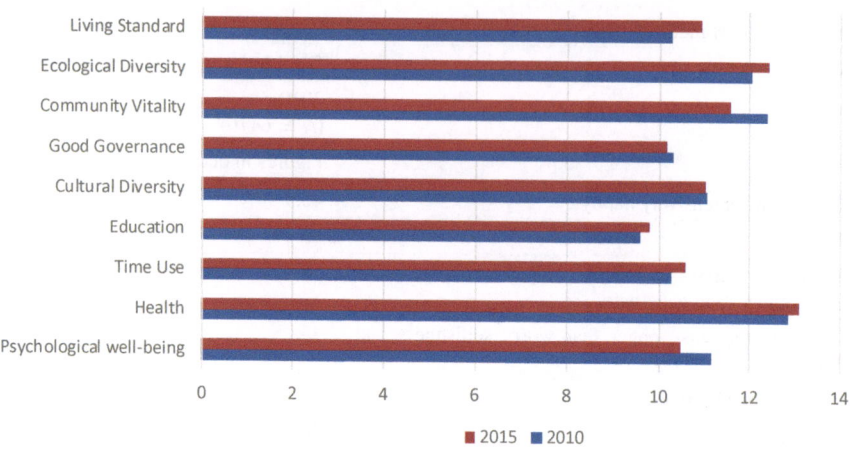

Fig. 4.4 Domain contribution in GNH index 2010–2015

than exports, and Bhutan is still largely dependent on India economically, which translates into a huge liquidity problem. Bhutan has prioritized three goals[40] which are: 1. Ending poverty in all its forms; 2. Urgent action to combat climate change and its impacts; and 3. Protect, restore and promote sustainable use of terrestrial ecosystems.

In 2018, the third general elections were held in Bhutan with two parties, viz., Druk Phuensum Tshogpa (DPT) and Druk Nyamrup Tshogpa (DNT). People's Democratic Party, the ruling party, could not get through the first election round which was held in September 2018. DNT won the final round of elections held in October 2018, which made Lotay Tshering, Bhutan's third prime minister since the adoption of the democratic constitution in 2008. DNT won 30 seats out of the available 47 assembly seats and DPT, with 17 seats, became the opposition party. It is interesting to note that in all three general elections held so far, the citizens have chosen a new party to lead rather than the incumbent, which indicates the resistance of voters and is an indicator of the maturation of democracy in Bhutan. This high political turnover is also evidence of the unhappiness with the ruling governments thus far. Dorji Penjore, chief researcher at the Center for Bhutan Studies and GNH Research, is of the opinion that party politics and democracy in Bhutan have caused a fall in psychological well-being and community vitality (Fig. 4.4) as reflected in the 2015 GNH survey report.[41] The GNH index of 2015 survey depicts a decrease in the public perception of government performance (Fig. 4.3).

Newly elected government led by Lotay Tshering has shown its serious concern over improving health and education well-being. He was the only practicing trained

---

[40] See RGOB (2018).

[41] See   https://www.washingtonpost.com/world/asia_pacific/in-tiny-bhutan-known-for-its-pursuit-of-happiness-democracy-brings-discontent/2018/10/17/05e43118-d229-11e8-a275-81c671a50422_story.html?noredirect=on&utm_term=.af67a6fd0a86 accessed on Oct 21, 2018.

urological surgeon in Bhutan and his concern for improving health well-being is applauded the citizens of Bhutan. On the weekends he visits the hospital and performs surgery which is applauded from all corners.[42] In order to improve the quality of teachers and motivate brilliant minds to opt for teaching as a career, Bhutan government has recommended remarkable increase in salary of teachers.[43] For some categories of teachers, it is around 100% increase. These initiatives by the current government in Bhutan shall go a long way in improving HWB and would help other countries to follow suit.

After taking office, the new prime minister endorsed the draft of the 12th five-year plan, which formulates strategies for July 1, 2018 to June 30, 2023. The objective of this plan is broadly: "Just, harmonious and sustainable society through enhanced decentralization."[44] The draft document provides strategic framework for the maximization of GNH (Fig. 4.5), in compliance with all broader policy frameworks—the constitution; king's addresses; Vision 2020; GNH strategy; GNH survey results; 11th Plan review; international and regional goals (SDGs, etc.); and stakeholder consultation. This framework is meant to provide guidance for all general public policy in Bhutan. Public policy direction and methods of measurement for achievement across performance indicators is detailed in the 12th five-year plan document. This document also provides the guidelines for assigning agency responsibility and role of

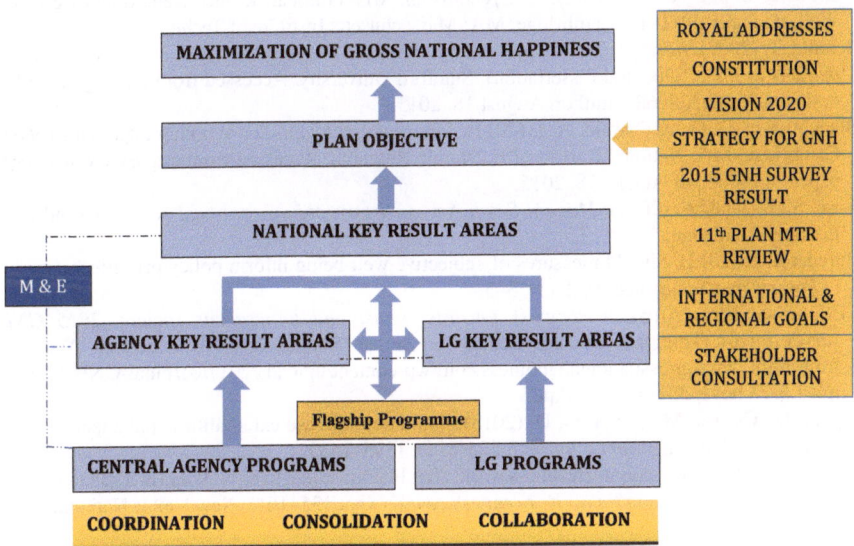

Fig. 4.5 Strategic framework (for maximising GNH)

---

[42] See a report by the telegraph https://www.telegraph.co.uk/news/2019/05/10/bhutan-prime-minister-spends-weekends-moonlighting-surgeon/.

[43] See https://www.weforum.org/agenda/2019/06/good-news-for-teachers-in-bhutan-the-government-is-doubling-their-pay/.

[44] See GNHC (2017).

the local government along with time lines for achieving the goals. Monitoring and evaluation loop between agency/local government programs and local Key Result Areas (KRAs) which are linked to national KRAs to help establish the relationship between planning, implementation, and execution.

It will be challenging for to the government to respond to the expectations of citizens and to improve life satisfaction for its people. The prime minister along with all his cabinet members, has a great responsibility in building those conditions and enabling the pursuit of GNH as enshrined in their constitution.

References

Adhikari, D. (2016). Healthcare and happiness in the Kingdom of Bhutan. *Singapore Medical Journal, 57*(3), 107–109. https://doi.org/10.11622/smedj.2016049.

Bajaj, M., & Kidwai, H. (2016). Human rights and education policy in South Asia. In K. Mundy, A. Green, R. Lingard, & A. Verger (Eds.), *Handbook of global education policy* (pp. 206–223). Hoboken, NJ: Wiley-Blackwell.

Basu, K. (2006). A note on management of state finances in West Bengal. In R. K. Sen & A. Dasgupta (Eds.), *Management of state finances* (pp. 209–219). New Delhi: Deep & Deep Publications.

Beath, A., Christia, F., & Enikolopov, R. (2012). *Winning hearts and minds through development: Evidence from a field experiment in Afghanistan.* MIT Political Science Department Research Working Paper 2011–14. Cambridge, MA: Massachusetts Institute of Technology.

Beteille, T. (2009). *Absenteeism, transfers and patronage: The political economy of teacher labor markets in India* (Doctoral dissertation). Stanford University. Accessed from http://gradworks. umi.com/33/82/3382684.html on August 18, 2015.

Blanchflower, D. G., & Oswald, A. J. (2011). *International happiness.* Working Paper No. 16668. Cambridge, MA: National Bureau of Economic Research. Accessed from http://www.nber.org/papers/w16668.pdf August 18, 2015.

Bose, S., & Jalal, A. (2004). *Modern South Asia—History, culture, political economy* (2nd ed.). London: Routledge.

Burchardt, T. (2013). Should measures of subjective well-being inform policy priorities? *Journal of Poverty and Social Justice, 21*(1), 3–5.

CBS, & GNHR. (2016). *A compass towards a just and harmonious society—2015 GNH survey report.* Thimphu, Bhutan: Centre for Bhutan Studies & GNH Research. Accessed from http://www.grossnationalhappiness.com/wp-content/uploads/2017/01/Final-GNH-Report-jp-21.3.17-ilovepdf-compressed.pdf.

Coffey, D., Geruso, M., & Spears, D. (2018). Sanitation, disease externalities, and anaemia: Evidence from Nepal. *Economic Journal, 128*(611), 1395–1432.

Das, G. (2002). A new emerging business world after liberalization. In N. N. Vohra & S. Bhattacharya (Eds.), *Looking back: India in the twentieth century* (pp. 135–161). New Delhi: National Book Trust.

Datta, A. (2013). Work, gender and social value. In M. Dutta (Ed.), *Gender and human development in Central and South Asia* (pp. 26–31). New Delhi: Pentagon Press.

De Neve, J., & Powdthavee, N. (2016, January 12). Income inequality makes whole countries less happy. *Harvard Business Review.* Retrieved from https://hbr.org/2016/01/income-inequality-makes-whole-countries-less-happy on 13.11.17.

Deaton, A. (2013). *The great escape: Health, wealth, and the origins of inequality.* Princeton, NJ: Princeton University Press.

Dirks, N. (2001). *Castes of mind: Colonialism and the making of modern India.* Princeton: Princeton University Press.

Dundar, H., Béteille, T., Riboud, M., & Deolalikar, A. (2014). *Student learning in South Asia: Challenges, opportunities, and policy priorities.* Washington, DC: International Bank for Reconstruction and Development/The World Bank.

Estes, R. J., & Zhou, H. (2014). A conceptual approach to the creation of public–private partnerships in social welfare. *International Journal of Social Welfare, 24*(4). https://doi.org/10.1111/ijsw.12142.

GFHR. (2001). *The 10/90 report on health research 2000.* Geneva: Global Forum for Health Research.

GIWPS. (2017). *Women, Peace and Security Index 2017-2018.* The Georgetown Institute for Women, Peace and Security. Washington, DC. USA accessed from https://giwps.georgetown.edu/wp-content/uploads/2017/10/WPS-Index-Report-2017-18.pdf.

GNHC. (2017). *12th five year plan (2018–2013).* Thimphu: Gross National Happiness Commission, Government of Bhutan. Accessed from https://www.gnhc.gov.bt/en/wp-content/uploads/2017/05/Finalized-Guideline.pdf.

Hsieh, C., & Klenow, P. J. (2009). Misallocation and manufacturing TFP in China and India. *Quarterly Journal of Economics, 124*(4), 1403–1448.

International Monetary Fund. (2004). *Bhutan: Poverty reduction strategy paper* (IMF Country Report No. 04/246). Washington, DC: IMF. Accessed from http://www.imf.org/external/pubs/ft/scr/2004/cr04246.pdf on August 18, 2015.

IPCC. (2007). *Climate change 2007: Impacts, adaptation and vulnerability.* Contribution of Working Group II to the Fourth Assessment Report of the Intergovernmental Panel on Climate Change. Cambridge: Cambridge University Press.

Jamil, I., Askvik, S., & Dhakal, T. N. (2013). *Understanding governance in South Asia.* New York: Springer. https://doi.org/10.1007/978-1-4614-7372-5_2.

Khanna, G., & Zimmermann, L. (2015). *Guns and butter? Fighting violence with the promise of development.* IZA Discussion Paper 9160. Bonn, Germany: Institute for the Study of Labor.

Larson, A. (2016). *Women and power: Mobilising around Afghanistan's elimination of violence against women law.* London: Overseas Development Institute.

Lateef, K. S. (2016). *Evolution of the World Bank's thinking on governance.* Background Paper World Development Report 2017—Governance and the Law. Accessed from http://pubdocs.worldbank.org/en/433301485539630301/WDR17-BP-Evolution-of-WB-Thinking-on-Governance.pdf.

Mahal, A. (2003). The distribution of public health subsidies in India. In A. S. Yazbeck & D. H. Peters (Eds.), *Health policy research in South Asia: Building capacity for reform* (pp. 33–63). *Human Development Network—Health, Nutrition, and Population Series.* Washington, DC: The World Bank.

Martin, R., Béteille, T., Li, Y., Mitra, P. K., & Newman, J. L. (2015). *Addressing inequality in South Asia.* Washington, DC: International Bank for Reconstruction and Development/The World Bank.

Muni, S. D. (1979). India and regionalism in South Asia: A political perspective. In B. Prasad (Ed.), *India's foreign policy: Studies in continuity and change* (pp. 105–124). New Delhi: Vikas Publishing House.

Nepali, R. K. (2009). *Democracy in South Asia.* Stockholm, Sweden: International Institute for Democracy and Electoral Assistance.

O'Neill, J., & Poddar, T. (2008). *Ten things for India to achieve its 2050 potential.* Global Economics Paper 169. Washington, DC: Goldman Sachs. Accessed from http://www.goldmansachs.com/our-hinking/archive/archive-pdfs/ten-things-india.pdf.

OPHI. (2018). *Global multidimensional poverty index 2018: The most detailed picture to date of the world's poorest people.* Oxford, UK: Oxford Poverty and Human Development Initiative, University of Oxford.

Peters, D. H., & Yazbeck, A. S. (2003). A framework for health policy research in South Asia. In A. S. Yazbeck & D. H. Peters (Eds.), *Health policy research in South Asia: Building capacity for reform* (pp. 23–30). *Human Development Network—Health, Nutrition, and Population Series.* Washington, DC: The World Bank.

Phuntsho, K. (2013). *The history of Bhutan*. India: Random House.

Planning Commission. (1999). *Bhutan 2020: A vision for peace, prosperity and happiness. Part II*. Thimphu: Planning Commission Secretariat, Royal Government of Bhutan. Accessed from http://www.gnhc.gov.bt/wp-content/uploads/2011/05/Bhutan2020_2.pdf on January 10, 2016.

Planning Commission. (2000). *Bhutan national human development report 2000—Gross national happiness and human development: Searching for common ground*. Thimphu: Planning Commission Secretariat, Royal Government of Bhutan. Accessed from http://hdr.undp.org/sites/default/files/bhutan_2000_en.pdf on January 10, 2016.

Planning Commission. (2002). *9th five-year-plan (2002–2007) main document*. Thimphu: Planning Commission Secretariat, Royal Government of Bhutan. Accessed from http://www.gnhc.gov.bt/wp-content/uploads/2011/04/5yp09_main.pdf on January 10, 2016.

Rangarajan, L. N. (Ed.). (1992). *Kautilya—The Arthashastra*. Gurgaon: Penguin Random House India.

RGOB. (2005). *Bhutan national human development report—The challenge of youth employment*. Thimphu: Royal Government of Bhutan. Accessed from http://hdr.undp.org/sites/default/files/bhutan_2005_en.pdf on January 10, 2016.

RGOB. (2018). *Sustainable development and happiness, Bhutan's voluntary national review report on the implementation of the 2030 agenda for sustainable development*. UN High Level Political Forum. Thimphu, Bhutan: Ministry of Finance, Royal Government of Bhutan. Accessed from https://www.gnhc.gov.bt/en/wp-content/uploads/2018/07/VNR_Bhutan_July2018.pdf.

Rosling, H. (2018). *Factfulness—Ten reasons we're wrong about the world—And why things are better than you think*. London: Hodder & Stoughton.

Rudolph, L. I., & Rudolph, S. H. (2001). Redoing the constitutional design: From an interventionist to a regulatory state. In A. Kohli (Ed.), *The success of India's democracy* (pp. 127–162). *Contemporary South Asia Series*. New York: Cambridge University Press.

Rutland, M. (1999). Bhutan—From the mediaeval to the millennium. *Journal of the Royal Society for Asian Affairs, 3*(3), 284–294.

Sadana, R., D'Souza, C., Hyder, A. A., & Chowdhury, A. M. R. (2004). Importance of health research in South Asia. *British Medicine Journal, 328*(7443), 826–830. https://doi.org/10.1136/bmj.328.7443.826. Accessed from https://www.ncbi.nlm.nih.gov/pmc/articles/PMC383385/.

Shrotryia, V. K. (2005). Perspectives on relevance of Gandhi for happiness and development. *Anasakti Darshan, International Journal of Non-Violence in Action, 1*(1), 92–103.

Shrotryia, V. K. (2006). Happiness and development—Public policy initiatives in the Kingdom of Bhutan. In Y. K. Ng & L. S. Ho (Eds.), *Happiness and public policy: Theory, case studies and implications*. Basingstoke: Palgrave Macmillan.

Shrotryia, V. K. (2009). Shift in the measures of quality of life viz-a-viz happiness: A study of Phongmey Gewog and Trashigang Town in Eastern Bhutan. In K. Ura & D. Penjore (Eds.), *Gross national happiness: Practice and measurement* (pp. 525–547). Thimphu: The Centre for Bhutan Studies.

Shrotryia, V. K. (2017). The history of well-being in South Asia. In R. J. Estes & M. J. Sirgy (Eds.), *The pursuit of human well-being—The untold global history* (pp. 349–380). International Handbooks on Quality of Life. Switzerland: Springer International Publishing.

Smith, A. (1984). *The theory of moral sentiments*. Indianapolis: Liberty Fund Inc.

Sreekumar, P. (2014). Development with diversity: Political philosophy of language endangerment in South Asia. *Economic & Political Weekly, 49*(1), 51–57.

Trading Economics. (2015). *World Bank indicators: South Asia—density & urbanization*. Accessed from http://www.tradingeconomics.com/south-asia/rural-population-growth-annual-percent-wb-data.html on August 18, 2015.

UNDP. (2013). *Human development report 2013: The rise of the South: Human progress in a diverse world*. United Nations Development Programme. New York: University Press.

UNDP. (2014). *Human development report 2014: Sustaining human progress: Reducing vulnerability and building resilience*. New York: United Nations Development Programme.

United Nations. (2001). Country presentation by the Royal Government of Bhutan. In *Third United Nations Conference on the Least Developed Countries (A/CONF.191/CP/16)*. Brussels: United Nations. Accessed from http://unctad.org/en/Docs/aconf191cp16bhu.en.pdf on August 18, 2015.

United Nations Millennium Project. (2005). *Investing in development: A practical plan to achieve the millennium development goals*. New York: United Nations Development Programme.

Ura, K., Alkire, S., Zangmo, T., & Wangdi, K. (2015). *Provisional findings of 2015 GNH survey*. Thimphu, Bhutan: Centre for Bhutan Studies & GNH Research.

Valente, C. (2011). *What did the Maoists ever do for us? Education and marriage of women exposed to civil conflict in Nepal*. Policy Research, Working Paper No. 5741. Washington, DC: World Bank. Accessed from http://elibrary.worldbank.org/doi/pdf/10.1596/1813-9450-5741 on August 18, 2015.

Von, T. A. (2007). *Indian summer: The secret history of the end of an empire*. London: Simon & Schuster.

Winkelmann, R., & Winkelmann, L. (1998). Why are the unemployed so unhappy? Evidence from panel data. *Economica, 65,* 1–15.

World Bank. (2011). *World development report 2012: Gender, equality and development*. Washington, DC: The World Bank.

World Bank. (2012). *World development report 2013: Jobs*. Washington, DC: The World Bank.

World Bank. (2013). *World development report 2014: Risk and opportunity—managing risk for development*. Washington, DC: The World Bank.

World Bank. (2015a). *World development report 2015: Mind, society, and behavior*. Washington, DC: The World Bank.

World Bank. (2015b). *Global monitoring report 2014/2015: Ending poverty and sharing prosperity*. Washington, DC: The World Bank.

World Bank. (2017). *World development report 2017—Governance and the law*. Washington, DC: The International Bank for Reconstruction and Development, The World Bank.

World Bank. (2018). *World development report 2018: Learning—To realize education's promise*. Washington, DC: The World Bank.

Yazbeck, A. S., & Peters, D. H. (2003). Overview. In A. S. Yazbeck & D. H. Peters (Eds.), *Health policy research in South Asia: Building capacity for reform* (pp. 3–21). *Human Development Network—Health, Nutrition, and Population Series*. Washington, DC: The World Bank.

Chapter 5
Conclusion and the Way Forward

*The ocean is the goal of all streams
and of the rain from the clouds,
yet it is never overflowing and never emptied:
so the* Dharma *is embraced by many millions of people,
yet it neither increases nor decreases.*
[Buddha][a]

Abstract This final chapter summarizes the book providing key takeaways. In addition to the key takeaways, a purposeful argument for public policy based on the priority of human well-being over conventional GDP has been built utilizing the experiences of the world, since the inception of GDP. The HWB developments in the field of academics as well as need for HWB-focused policy shift has been narrated in brief. Policies focusing on building superior education systems and sustainable health systems are strongly suggested. As South Asia falls under the "developing" category, heavy migration from rural to urban areas is evident. In that context, a vision for building happy cities is required which has been briefed in the following chapter. The use of technology specially for improving governance has been highlighted and discussion around technological policies has been incorporated wherever considered appropriate. This chapter concludes with an analysis of comparative strengths, weaknesses, opportunities, and threats emphasized for guiding future policy direction.

Keywords Human well-being · South Asia · GDP · Technology · Happy cities · Governance · Education · Health

5.1 Introduction

Human well-being should ideally be the primary target of all policies in a state—internal or external. In order to rule successfully, the government must ensure that policies are effectively communicated and positively affect the well-being of each citizen. General living conditions across world have improved, as is the case in South

---

[a]see Carus 1995, p. LXI.4.

© Springer Nature Switzerland AG 2020
V. K. Shrotryia, *Human Well-Being and Policy in South Asia*, Human Well-Being
Research and Policy Making, https://doi.org/10.1007/978-3-030-33270-9_5

Asia. The speed and density of progress made in the domain of HWB, are highlighted when the geography of this region is compared with other parts of the world. The legacy of the British Raj in most part of South Asia region, has been damaging to development to a large extent. Two centuries of primarily British colonial rule left the region economically bankrupt with divided and feudalistic mindset. Basic infrastructure (railways, roads, bridges, etc.) which the British required to practice trade, was created and maintained during the colonial period. Hospitals and schools run by missionaries during the colonial period made impacts throughout the South Asian population. The young minds were shaped by the education that was provided with an intent to restrict them to get white collar jobs. Thinking, as a mental activity, was not something that was thought of being a requirement of youth during the period of colonial rule as it engulfed the brains of the majority of youth. The ancient education system for which South Asia was once applauded across the world was systematically ruined by colonization; of the effects of which the region is still suffering from.

Maddison mentions that pre-independence India (including Bangladesh and Pakistan) and China were both had strong economies until 1870; they contributed about two-thirds of the world's GDP. He further states: "Moghul India had a bigger industry than any other country which became a European colony, and was unique in being an industrial exporter in pre-colonial times. A large part of this industry was destroyed as a consequence of British rule" (Maddison, 1995, p. 115). In the 16th century, on an average, Indians had relatively higher incomes and lower taxation rates than their counterparts elsewhere in the world. Gold, diamonds, fine shawls, spices, and opium were commonly sold in the markets during that period (Von, 2007). Around the 18th century and before foreign colonization, the general economic well-being of the residents in this part of the world was much better than that of the residents in other parts of the world.

The last 70 years of progress in the region has primarily witnessed economic growth. Yet, the impact of economic growth leading towards human development (or holistic development) has been contentious across the region (also see Shrotryia, 2017). Inequality created by economic growth or development (Piketty, 2014) is seen across the region. Economic development entails more than the acquisition of, and addition to wealth. The distribution of wealth is equally important for sustainable HWB and determining the best policies for the equitable distribution of wealth is extremely difficult. Equitable distribution of resources and holistic development remains a significant challenge for the region.

As discussed so far, income, health, education, and governance have all significantly impacted HWB. Expected outcomes have not been achieved. And it is also seen that to a greater extent the priorities were misplaced. The privatization of education at all levels has provided some short-term solutions which have more long-term implications, and India in particular has started paying price for that. In terms of healthcare, privatization has resulted in more importance being placed on profit rather than on quality care. Profiteering is observed as a major concern for private hospitals which are exploiting patients. Government machinery involved in the delivery of services and public outreach is primarily motivated by its own selfish ends. Collectivism which once reflected the social fabric of South Asia is evolving into individualism. It is rather impossible to reason whether it is cyclic or driven by the visible set indicators. Or it has happened under the influence of some motivated international agencies. Only time will be able to answer it in future. Yet HWB has to improve, both physically and mentally, extrinsically and intrinsically. South Asia's potential is unparalleled in terms of the adaptability of its population. Caused by the dominance of working-class age, the region enjoys demographic dividend, which has to be addressed by providing gainful employment opportunities. South Asia would have to evolve ways to capitalize on the strength of its population and their earning abilities so that the dividend does not turn into deficit.

This chapter is designed to summarize the development that indicators reflect so far and to suggest a policy framework for the future.

5.2 Summarized Outcome

The South Asian region is known for its diversity as it is multicultural, multilingual, and multi-geographical. The eight countries that are studied in this monograph each have strengths and weaknesses of different kinds and severities. On one side South Asia contains the second most populated country of the world (India), while on the other side, it also has some of the least populated countries (the Maldives and Bhutan). Out of the eight countries, four are Muslim (Afghanistan, Bangladesh, the Maldives, and Pakistan), two are Buddhist (Bhutan and Sri Lanka), one is Hindu (Nepal), and one is secular (India). This diversity has its positives as well as its negatives. South Asia is Indo-centric as around three-fourths of the population lives in India and two of the countries (Pakistan and Bangladesh) formed from land that was once India. This region occupies less than 4% of the world's land mass yet houses around 24% of the world population. Around two-third of the population of this region still lives in villages, though in the last 27 years around 6% of the population moved from rural to urban areas. Bhutan and Nepal which had the lowest urban population in the region in 1991, have improved much faster than other countries in South Asia in changing that composition. Bhutan has largest population living in urban areas at around 40%, whereas more than 81% of Sri Lankans still live in rural villages. The smallest in land area and population, the Maldives, only has around 300 km^2 of land (0.0063%) and houses around just 0.02% of the South Asian population. Time series data of Afghanistan, the Maldives and Bhutan is sparse, though for last two decades it is organized.

Over the past two decades, South Asia has experienced strong economic growth. During 1991–2017, the GDP per capita of South Asia (at current USD) grew by around 5.5 times which is much faster than world GDP per capita growth (3.1 times). Bhutan has grown the fastest, followed by India, whereas Pakistan has grown the slowest. As per the preliminary report of the Multidimensional Poverty Index (MPI) 2018, Afghanistan is the poorest country followed by Pakistan; and the Maldives is the richest in the region followed by India. MPI does not include Sri Lanka, otherwise Sri Lanka would have ranked slightly below the Maldives and above India. Overall, economically this region has progressed very well.

This region now has improved health indicators and has almost reached world standards in terms of average life expectancy. People in the Maldives live much longer than their counterparts in other parts of South Asia and Afghans have the lowest life expectancy. However, Bhutan, Nepal, and Afghanistan have improved life expectancy during the last three decades, at a much faster rate than other countries of the region. The Maldives and Sri Lanka have been able to significantly reduce the infant mortality rate. They also have much better hospital coverage for their population, the available data on hospital beds and the availability of physicians in the Maldives and Sri Lanka reflects much higher levels of health care as compared to their South Asian counterparts. In 2015, Nepal and Afghanistan spent more than 10% of their GDP on health, which has resulted in some improvements in their health parameters. The out-of-pocket household expense share on healthcare in Afghanistan is the highest in the region. South Asian households spend much more on health expenses than their counterparts in any other region of the world. In the majority of the region, health facilities are privatized meaning that a myriad of different types of clinics and health centers can provide healthcare. The role of NGOs and philanthropies is also remarkable in most parts of the region.

Among all the countries of the region, Bhutan has been allocating greater share of its GDP towards education, which has had a clear positive effect on indicators. The absence of comparable time-series data on literacy rates, teachers at different levels etc. has certainly been a hurdle to reach to any conclusive conclusions, yet what is reflected through the available data is that there has been a gradual improvement in literacy levels of all the countries in the region. The Maldives and Sri Lanka have excellent literacy rates which are both above 90%; Afghanistan and Bangladesh are the laggards. Improvements in expected years of schooling indicate future improvement in terms of literacy levels. As education parameters improve, more people become job seekers and correspondingly employment opportunities are not created, resulting in increase in unemployment. This is prevalent across all of South Asia. Though employment opportunities are constantly being created, they are not sufficient enough to absorb the large number of youths leaving the college system. However, initiatives of different governments in the region to encourage youth to take up entrepreneurship are reaping good fruits. The World Bank (2019) reports, "The first start-up for business process outsourcing in India got appeared in 2002 and by 2012, around 2.8 million people were employed in this industry" (p. 73). While there has been sizeable job creation in some ICT related services, primarily in India, large number of jobs created in the services sector over the past few decades, have been in traditional low value-added services, where informality and vulnerable forms of employment are often dominant (ILO 2018: 22).

Access to education, at different levels, by all the countries of the region, has been handled well so far but quality is the most serious current concern. While the gross enrolment ratio is on the gradual rise, quality is not relatively improving. Meaning that while more children are being educated, the quality of that education has not kept pace with modern trends. More than unemployment, employability is a concern. The challenge is to provide vocational education and skill development programs so that employability can be improved.

Income, health, and education are the key variables for HDI. Sri Lanka and the Maldives are ranked as high human development countries whereas Afghanistan is ranked very poorly on the list of low human development countries. All others South Asian countries fall in the middle range. Around 96% of the population is living in the countries ranked (0–1) between 0.56 (Pakistan) and 0.64 (India) in HDI, meaning that they are at the medium human development level.

South Asia suffers from strong governance deficit which has been eating up much of its resources. Afghanistan ranks the poorest in terms of worldwide governance indicators and Bhutan ranks the highest in the region. In terms of the perception of corruption, as tracked by Transparency International, the same trend is observed. Though Sri Lanka and the Maldives have much better positions in HDI and other social indicators (such as education and healthcare), they are still not best in terms of governance parameters. Living conditions in Bangladesh, Pakistan, and Nepal need much more improvement as compared to other countries. As per the Women, Peace, and Security Index, living conditions in Afghanistan are the worst across the region, though there have been lots of improvements which have been previously examined in the book. Nepal has the best position on the Women, Peace, and Security Index as compared to other countries, followed by Sri Lanka.

The data on happiness levels as given in the World Happiness Report published since 2012, remains the most extensive and consistent published dataset. It does not include the Maldives however. As of 2018, Pakistan is the happiest nation in the region, followed by Bhutan; Afghanistan unsurprisingly has the lowest happiness rank in the region. The changes during 2012–2017 show that while in Sri Lanka, Pakistan, and Nepal, happiness levels have improved, yet in all other parts of the region there is a decline in happiness levels. It is surprising to note that although on most of the HWB indicators (as discussed in this monograph) Pakistan is not in the league of front runners, yet in the WHR it is named as happiest country from the region.

Examining the region's demographic profile and data related to income, poverty, health, education, and governance—which are considered to be the composite indicators for drawing the status of HWB in this book—provides us several key takeaways as follows:

a. More than two-thirds of the population lives in villages across the region, but living in villages is not a precondition to having low human well-being (e.g., Sri Lanka has around 81% of its population residing in villages, yet it has one of the best profiles on well-being).
b. Countries (the Maldives, Sri Lanka, and Bhutan) which have the highest standards in income, health, and education contain less than 2% of the population in the region. This leads us to assume that it is much easier to more efficiently manage small nations and assure their well-being, as government policies are easily monitored and the resources are more appropriately apportioned.
c. Having high standards in education and health does not guarantee high levels of governance, such as in the Maldives and Sri Lanka.

d. Containing three-fourths of the population in the region, India has improved poverty standards hugely in the last two decades and now has one of the lowest index values in global Multidimensional Poverty Index (just above the Maldives), a much better ranking as compared to other countries in the region. (Sri Lanka was not included in the MPI).

e. Government expenditure on health (excepting Afghanistan and Nepal) and education across the region is very low. On the contrary, individualout-of-pocket health-related expense of South Asian countries are the highest in the world. This imbalance is a significant negative strain on HWB.

f. Political strength and corruption significantly contribute overall governance indicators (Afghanistan, the Maldives, Pakistan, Nepal, and Bangladesh).

g. Size of the country negatively correlated to the effectiveness of administration which is reflected through indicators (The Maldives, Sri Lanka and Bhutan). The density of population is much better in these South Asian countries.

h. Data on happiness levels (Gallup World Poll as used in the World Happiness Report) does not significantly correlate with the social indicators like health, education, and governance.

i. Overall, the South Asian region has grown much better economically as compared to other analyzed indicators.

j. The focus on economic growth has not consequentially resulted in relative improvements in health, education, and governance indicators or general HWB.

With these takeaways in mind, the need for a policy shift away from focusing on economic growth towards one which focuses on HWB as a composite outcome is necessary. Hence the next part of this chapter examines developments across the globe on GDP and develops a strong case for a shift in the policy.

5.3   GDP Vis-à-Vis Human Well-Being: An Agenda for Future Policy

National progress has historically been judged solely by development in the economic sphere. The size of an economy and the level of development are predominantly driven by national income, termed Gross Domestic Product (or GDP). GDP was first introduced by Kuznets (1934) with an extensive account of national income during 1929–32. Paul Samuelson and William D. Nordhaus stated: "While the GDP and the rest of the national income accounts may seem to be arcane concepts, they are truly among the great inventions of the 20th century."[1] Weitzman (1976) believed that Net Domestic Product (NDP) can be regarded as a proxy for national welfare in the sense that it is proportional to the present discounted value of all future consumption. This belief did not gain many followers.

---

[1] See January 2000 issue of Survey of Current Business, page 6 available at: https://fraser.stlouisfed.org/files/docs/publications/SCB/pages/2000-2004/35260_2000-2004.pdf retrieved on September 13, 2018.

These economists never imagined that nations would use GDP as a basis for all their policies and practices. Much less that they would primarily concentrate on growth indicators surrounding GDP and measure the progress of nations by this standard of measurement. Economists and psychologists have discussed at length the fact that improvements in GDP do not translate into enhanced life satisfaction at length for people.[2] In the United States, the preamble to the Declaration of Independence lists life, liberty, and the pursuit of happiness as core rights which were the cornerstone upon which American democracy was built. Yet it is difficult to infer a straightforward relationship between government's objectives and human happiness. Whether human happiness can and should be the primary goal of a government, has long been debated (Sgroi, Hills, O'Donnell, Oswald, & Proto, 2017, p. 10). *The Progress Paradox* as coined by Easterbrook (2003) provides ample evidence that though physical infrastructure and the standard of living have improved in both the United States and Europe over the last 500 years, the life satisfaction or happiness of the people have not improved.

The focus of politics and policies, world over, has remained preferential towards the wealthy. As one of the Oxford Briefing papers mentions, economic inequality is increasing in most countries, increasing government policies that advance the interest of the rich. The polling results from Spain, Brazil, India, South Africa, the UK, and the US show that the majority in these countries believe that the legal and regulatory systems in their countries are crafted for the benefit of the rich (Oxfam, 2014). This has been a major cause of inequality interrupting HWB, though in aggregate terms, it reflects the good of the economy. The benefit of economic growth does not reach to the underprivileged strata of society in proportion to its benefits reaching to the rich. Economic growth also causes inappropriate distribution of wealth which does not result in corresponding improvements in HWB. The OECD and IMF[3] have also expressed their reservations and feel that inequality increases instability and damages economic growth. "A fifth of the world's population earns just 2% of global income. The richest 20% by contrast earn 74% of the world's income… in the advanced economies, inequality is higher than it was 20 years ago" (Jackson, 2009, p. 5). Such inequalities might reach a record high in 2020 (Wilkinson & Pickett, 2009).

All across the globe, the physical standard of living has improved manifold, yet the public's perception towards their life has often not improved *pari passu*. Physical infrastructure has been transformed to provide comforts of the so-called "good life," yet it has added community and social problems rather than adding to HWB. The gap between rich and the poor has exponentially increased all across the globe, all types of value (human) erosion is happening; consumerism is prevalent and materialism

---

[2] See Blanchflower and Oswald (2004), Cobb, Gary, Goodman, and Mathis (1999), Costanza, Hart, Posner, and Talbert (2009), Coyle (2014), Diener and Seligman (2004), Easterlin (1974, 1995, 2001), Frey and Stutzer (2002), Goossens, Makipaa, Philipp, and Isabel (2007), Helliwell (2003), Jackson (2006, 2009), Jebb, Tay, Diener, and Oishi (2018), van den Bergh (2007, 2009), Layard (2006), MaxNeef (1995), Nordhaus and Tobin (1973), Posner and Costanza (2011), Sen (1976, 1979), Stiglitz, Sen, and Fitoussi (2010), and many others.

[3] As mentioned in Ostry, Berg, and Tsangarides (2014).

has penetrated into public psyches. Individuals are often judged solely based on the physical wealth they possess. Though many nations are becoming more economically developed, richer, and more independent, the problems such as work-life conflict, discrimination, crime, depression, environmental imbalance, social alienations, etc., are on the rise.

The last decade of the 20th century witnessed the emergence and popularity of the Human Development Index (HDI) as an alternative to compare different national indicators. As the index analyzes economic as well as social development, it has been recognized as a better tool to help formulate effective public policy through improving health and education infrastructure. Better health and education standards strengthen human competence and empower individuals to create their own choices. Public policy needs to concentrate on developing better social infrastructure which will simultaneously work to improve economic indicators.

Bhutan, one of the smallest countries in the South Asian region, has been practicing a development philosophy based on the premise of well-being, defined as Gross National Happiness (GNH). It wasn't until early 2008 that this tiny kingdom became a parliamentary democracy. However, Bhutan was using GNH to influence policy as early as 1973. There have been persistent global efforts to popularize the concept of GNH and to advocate on the importance of happiness in policy framework. Wikiquote defines GHN as "an indicator and concept that measures quality of life or social progress in more holistic and psychological terms than only the economic indicator of Gross Domestic Product (GDP)."[4] As mentioned in one of Bhutan's national human development reports (see Planning Commission, 2000, p. 20), "pursuit of GNH calls for a multi-dimensional approach to development that seeks to maintain harmony and balance between economic forces, environmental preservation, cultural and spiritual values; and good governance. These four priorities are termed as the four pillars of GNH".[5]

In 2010, Joseph Stiglitz visited Bhutan to address policymakers, bureaucrats, and development agents. The focus of his address was on shifting from GDP to well-being, as he also critically argued in a report by the Commission on the Measurement of Economic Performance and Social Progress of which he was the chair. This commission was initiated by the president of the French Republic, Nicholas Sarkozy, in February 2008 after he felt dissatisfied with the state of statistical information available about the economy and societal happiness. The mandate of the Commission was to identify the limits of GDP as an indicator of economic performance and social progress; to consider what additional information might be required for the production of more relevant indicators of social progress; to assess the feasibility of alternative measurement tools; and to discuss how to present the statistical information in an appropriate way. The Commission members conducted research on social capital, happiness, and health and mental well-being.

---

[4]See https://en.wikiquote.org/wiki/Gross_national_happiness.

[5]A detailed note on Bhutan's practice of GNH, its practice and reflection through action oriented public policy has been discussed in an Annexure in Chap. 4.

The report, also known as the Sarkozy Report, made a strong case that it is time for our measurement system to shift its emphasis from measuring economic production to measuring people's well-being. Further, the Sarkozy Report also suggested that the measures of well-being should be analyzed in a context of sustainability. The Commission gave five recommendations apart from looking at the well-being spectrum, which are: 1. when evaluating material well-being, look at income and consumption rather than production, 2. emphasize the household perspective, 3. consider income and consumption jointly with wealth, 4. give more prominence to the distribution of income, consumption, and wealth, and, 5. broaden income measures to non-market activities.

Easterlin (1974) was perhaps the first economist of the modern era who studied the relationship between happiness and economic outcome which culminated into a paradox known as the Easterlin Paradox. The Easterlin Paradox states that a rise in income does not result in a similar rise in happiness. The Easterlin Paradox was published long before the Sarkozy report. Similarly, in the UK, the New Economic Foundation (NEF), started developing the Happy Planet Index (HPI) which looked at life satisfaction, life expectancy, and ecological footprints. Apart from the HPI, the NEF also develops national accounts of well-being (as advocated by Daniel Kahneman) which includes measures of personal, social, and emotional well-being.

In 2006, the British Broadcasting Corporation (BBC) carried out a survey on happiness which reported that 47% respondents recognized family relationships as much more important for their own happiness and wellbeing, only 8% ranked money and financial status highest in importance. It concluded by stating that increase in reported life satisfaction is only weakly correlated with rising income which is termed the "wellbeing paradox" (Jackson, 2006, p. 16). Princeton University Press, published "The politics of happiness-what government can learn from the new research on well-being" by Derek Bok in 2010. Based on global research, this book makes a strong case for policymakers to prioritize well-being over excessive focus on the market economy (Bok, 2010). Alex Michalos (known for his work on the Canadian Index of Well-being), categorically mentions that:

> The economists messed everything up, the main barrier to getting progress has been that statistical agencies around the world are run by economists and statisticians and they are not people who are comfortable with human beings. The fundamental national measure they employ tells us a good deal about the economy but almost nothing about the specific things in our lives that really matter.[6]

Are we ready to shift our focus towards well-being encompassing every sense of the term rather than only using it through the window of economic parameters? This is a major challenge facing the state and policymakers.

It was July 19, 2011 when 68 nations joined Bhutan in support of its resolution titled "Happiness: Towards a holistic approach to development" for adoption by the United Nations. The UN General Assembly adopted this resolution which recognized

---

[6]Cited by Jon Gertner in an article published in *New York Times Magazine* on May 10, 2010, entitled "The Rise and Fall of the GDP" available at http://www.glaserprogress.org/program_areas/pdf/The_Rise_and_Fall_of_the_GDP_-_Jon_Gertner_NYT_051010.pdf.

happiness as a fundamental human goal and emphasized a more inclusive, equitable, and balanced approach to economic growth that promotes the happiness and well-being of all. The resolution stated: "The GDP indicator by nature was not designed to and does not adequately reflects the happiness and wellbeing of people in a country."[7] This resolution mandated that member nations take steps towards realizing a development paradigm with integrating economic, social, and environmental objectives going beyond GDP-based development. The resolution invited member states "to pursue the elaboration of additional measures that better capture the importance of the pursuit of happiness and well-being in development with a view to guiding their public policies."[8]

Taking its cue from this resolution, the UN hosted its first high-level meeting on April 2, 2012 on the theme of "Happiness and Well-being: Defining a New Economic Paradigm." The then prime minister of Bhutan, Jigme Y. Thinley, was the driving force behind the 2012 UN meeting. This historical meeting was attended by select heads of state, ministers, Nobel laureates, eminent economists, scholars, and spiritual and civil society leaders from around the world. The UN Secretary General Ban Ki Moon said: "We need a new economic paradigm that recognizes the parity between the three pillars of sustainable development. Social, economic and environmental well-beings are indivisible. Together they define gross global happiness."[9] On June 28, 2012 all of the 193 member-states of the UN General Assembly unanimously adopted UN Resolution 66/281 and decided to observe March 20th as International Day of Happiness or International Happiness Day.

The former president of India, A. P. J. Abdul Kalam, agreed that GDP does not reflect improvements in quality of life. He stated:

> While we are happy that our economy is in an ascending phase and our GDP has been growing at as high as 9% per annum, it is evident that the economic growth is not fully reflected in the quality of life of a large number of people, particularly in rural areas and even in urban areas. Hence, we have evolved what is called a National Prosperity Index (NPI), which is a summation of (a) annual growth rate of GDP; (b) improvement in quality of life of people, particularly those living below the poverty line: and (c) the adoption of a value system derived from our civilizational heritage in every walk of life which is unique to India. That is NPI = a+b+c. Particularly, 'b' is a function of availability of housing, good water, nutrition, proper sanitation, quality education, quality health care and employment potential, and 'c' is a function of promoting the joint family system, creation of a spirit of working together, leading a righteous way of life, removing social inequities, and above all promoting a conflict-free, harmonious society. This will be indicated by peace in families and communities, reduction in corruption index, reduction in court cases, elimination of violence against children and women, and the absence of communal tensions. There should be progressive reduction in the number of people living below the poverty line leading to this number becoming near zero by 2020. All our efforts at improving the national economic performance should be guided by the National prosperity Index of the nation at any point of time. (Abdul Kalam, 2012, p. 53)

---

[7]See https://news.un.org/en/story/2011/07/382052.

[8]See Footnote 7.

[9]See Footnote 7.

Most of the outcomes mentioned in this monograph are parts of the larger con-struct of HWB. In the current era of market force dominance and enormous capital flows, focus on HWB in public policy should be viewed as a transformational ini-tiative. The last two decades have produced voluminous literature on the different aspects of happiness, human well-being, quality of life, etc., through a myriad of aca-demic and experiential research. Alternative approaches to GDP in order to measure progress and development are being studied and developed in all parts of the world, so future generations will be able to view societies from more holistic perspectives and parameters.

As far back as 1776, Adam Smith strongly believed that material possessions do not provide happiness, even though most of mankind was relentlessly involved in the struggle to acquire more wealth and the social disgrace of not being able to acquire more was the greatest pain of being poor (Smith, 1984). On the other hand, agencies like the World Bank believe that "nothing besides long-term high rate of GDP growth, can solve the world's poverty problem" (World Bank, 2008). Kuznets himself stated that the welfare of a nation can hardly be seen from a measure of national income.[10] In the given conditions, it is difficult to understand the view of the World Bank. But what is not difficult to understand is that human well-being is an end and GDP a mean to that end, the reversal of this fact will ruin the future of public policy.

Growth that is merely financial, development that is lopsided, progress that is based only on quantification, will not lead us towards a better future. It is long over-due that happiness is given priority over generally quantifiable measures. Human happiness and well-being should be the sole target of public policy, financial indi-cators will organically improve as well-being does. Around the beginning of this century Polly Toynbee wrote in The Guardian: "When God died, GDP took over and economists became the new high priests. That has been the story of the last century."[11] The 21st century should be the century which goes down in history as an era targeting HWB and happiness over economic development.

5.4   Policy Interventions in South Asia

As the constituent nations of South Asia are progressing, their policy framework is becoming more organized. The planning structure has been very similar across nations, i.e., most of them followed five-year plans which were focused on clearly identified priorities, and investments were made accordingly. Public expenditure had country specific and situation specific priority. For most policy formation, govern-ments were dependent on the bureaucrats who were responsible for helping and

---

[10]See https://www.nytimes.com/2011/10/09/opinion/sunday/gdp-doesnt-measure-happiness.html accessed on October 24, 2018.

[11]See https://www.theguardian.com/politics/2003/mar/07/society.politicalcolumnists accessed on October 28, 2018.

advising the government select national priorities. The political leadership takes the call on the basis of national priority, matching with its election manifesto and demand. The developmental progress in other world regions and larger global priorities have helped shape policy framework in the South Asian region, such as resolutions from the UN or other international organizations or/and funding agencies. Membership to international organizations, bilateral and multilateral agreements, global resolutions, etc., mandates which countries enjoy certain sanctions—fund allocations for given causes—to enact corresponding policy to improve global well-being. Such as in 2000 when the Millennium Development Goals (MDGs) were established by the UN to advance societal development goals at national level, meaning that the recipient countries were then committed these goals in their policy frameworks. When MDGs were transformed into SDGs in 2015, similar commitments were expected and were reflected through national policies. Removal of hunger, poverty, and inequality; ensuring inclusive and equitable education; ensuring good health and well-being; etc., have been some the goals which UN member countries have implemented through their related policies. Progress is maintained through periodic monitoring to make sure that these targets are being achieved at a steady pace by member countries.

The government often seeks policy advice from internal governmental institutions as well as from prominent think tanks, which have proliferated and influenced civil society. These institutions and civil society activists have been able to develop a mechanism for getting their voices heard. But, scholarship in South Asia has not paid the required attention to the dimension of public policy where they are involved in the public policy discourses (Mathur, 2013, p. 75). Economically, South Asia has progressed well and developed resources for investing in the social sector but somehow these resources cannot be effectively allocated and implemented to improve the various indicators. Health indicators have more positively improved as compared to education, which still needs serious improvement.

A national government level formal system needs to be devised in all countries of the region. Such system has to be holistic in its approach and should be able to engage all stakeholders. A model as suggested by Estes and Zhou (2014) provides a good background for adoption by making modifications looking at the country requirements. Public-private partnerships, as practiced in some cases in India, are a good beginning for sharing responsibility which allows private entrepreneurs to maintain a sense of ownership while providing the government with increased resources. NGOs are also involved in the process of delivering social goods to the public, which needs to be encouraged but at the same time regulated. The policy focus of different governments in the region has been highlighted in Chap. 3 followed by a detailed discussion on concerning problems and priorities in Chap. 4.

There is a lot to learn from Bhutan, which has not only been including happiness in their policies but is also implementing policies in such a way that a progress check is made at every level (also see Shrotryia, 2017). Governance indicators in Bhutan are the highest in the region, as discussed previously in this monograph. The public policy framework thus should have contributions from civil society, feedback from households, and the opinion of experts and interest groups in order to increase policy effectiveness. This has started happening at some levels through the use of technology that is inviting feedback from the public. MyGov is an excellent example of this, developed by the government of India, to engage with the public using technology. This sounds quite promising, but the problem is that the region has not yet created a healthy environment where free and fair opinions are exchanged for the good of policy direction. And that is where education should be blamed and improved. The involvement of stakeholders and emphasis on KRAs at different levels of governance in Bhutan's strategic plan is a good example.

5.5 On Education and Health

The education system as designed by Thomas Babington Macaulay in the mid-19th century for India (which included present-day Pakistan and Bangladesh) was aimed to create office clerks and blue-collar workers. The other countries of the region were also influenced by that system of education. The current educational system still suffers from that legacy. The mindset of Macaulay's educational policies has been ingrained into much of the population and negatively affecting the thinking and creative faculties of modern students. The education system needs thorough review if India is to improve their educational indicators. Rote learning dominates in most schools across South Asia, which makes students literate enough to get white-collar jobs but not educated enough to make sensible and progressive contributions to their nation. Education is such an important domain for development that all other development indicators are compromised if the educational system is poor and more so if it produces masses that are not highly employable. So, the primary focus of public policy across South Asia should be to improve the education system and to strengthen institutions of higher learning. The target of improving the gross enrolment ratio must be fully complemented with a focus on the quality of education at all levels.

It is important to note that all the countries of the region have utilized private sector investments towards education through philanthropy, though it has become a business in many cases. Private sector investment in education has caused exponential growth in schools, colleges, and universities and it is becoming a challenge for countries to regulate these institutions in order to maintain quality.

The health sector requires huge investments. The availability of doctors is a key issue for the region. The Maldives and Nepal boasts of a much better status in terms of the availability of physicians, but all other countries of the region suffer from shortage of qualified doctors. The focus of policy should be to first create good institutions which provide quality medical education and then to nurture students to become good doctors. Surprisingly, the number of aspiring students who choose their career after secondary levels are more inclined to pursue engineering than the medical field. Low attendance rates to medical schools are largely affected by the return on investment in terms of time on education spent, which in case of engineering is much lower. The choice of career is majorly influenced by factors like—number of years spent in study, nature of efforts that are required, and relatively better job placement. The higher cost of medical education is also one of the reasons why it is less popular than other fields. STEM (Science, Technology, Engineering, and Mathematics) is a preferred choice for aspiring professionals as compared to medical education due to better perceived opportunities, less time in school, and higher pay packages. This will cause a significant problem for almost entire region but more for India, because of demand-supply gap. The medical profession is subservient to market forces and experiences intense competition to earn more money as compared to the feeling of serving the society. The major cause of these problems has been the absence of good medical institutions for responding to the size of regional population. This must be addressed through interventions in policy and by investing more in building quality medical education institutions which are fully supported by the government.

The Public-Private Development Mix Model (Estes & Zhou, 2014) offers a practical solution to the problem of the availability of funds for carrying out welfare measures. Involvement of private entrepreneurs and good corporate citizens in sharing state responsibility through Public-Private Partnership mode should be encouraged. More so for the countries in the South Asian region, which are facing challenges directly to want of funds. As mentioned in Chap. 3, government expenditure on social infrastructure across South Asia region is too low which is caused by two important factors: one, the social sector is not a priority area for government planning as it does not provide a visible return in the short term; two, the lack of financial resources and the pressing need to spend on other sectors which seem more urgent and assure a visible return. Corporate Social Responsibility (CSR), which is a mix of state, market, and civil society, is playing an important role in India. The government had made it mandatory for corporations to share 2% of their profit to go towards building facilitating infrastructure and sharing the responsibility of the state in running socially beneficial projects. Much of the expense out of the CSR budget is allocated to education, health, environment, and governance.

5.6 On Building Happy Cities

One of the reports of the World Economic Forum[12] identified four key issues that millennials in South Asia have to confront. They are as follows: 1. Equitable growth; 2. Livable and sustainable cities; 3. Education, employment, and entrepreneurship; and 4. Regional collaboration. All of these issues are important and must find a place in the policy for assuring a prosperous future for South Asia. For urban planning and for assuring better HWB, there are important interventions to be made by urban planners, the state, architects, and civil society. At a time when a population shift from rural to urban areas is happening at a rapid pace across the region, urban planning becomes all the more important. Yet it is challenging to discuss, design,

---

[12]See https://www.weforum.org/agenda/2016/10/top-issues-for-south-asia-millennials/ retrieved on October 21, 2016.

and develop cities with the kind of infrastructural support that can ease living and provide comfortable stay with easy accessibility for amenities.

The use of technology and artificial intelligence can help designers propose a system which is technologically advanced and is compatible with modern climate change conditions. Green and clean technologies should find an appropriate place in the cities of the future. In the times of digital assistants like Alexa, Cortana, Siri, and Google Now, the houses and cities must be made smart-home compatible so that the users of tomorrow find it convenient to adapt. In 2013, Charles Montgomery wrote a book entitled *Happy city: Transforming our lives through urban design* which restarted the debate on building cities where happiness of residents is a priority (Montgomery, 2013). This book contains strong narratives detailing experiences of happiness and defends the science of happiness and its relationship with urban planning.

Rural urban migration, which is a sign of development, has to be managed through providing urban amenities to rural areas as visualized and proposed by former Indian President Abdul Kalam in the name of PURA.[13] PURA needs to be given serious thought so that the burden on urban cities is reduced. Better educational facilities and health infrastructure has to be prioritized so that the villages are livable and the primary conditions of living are improved. Road connectivity, electricity and water, sanitation, and sewerage are some such areas which have to be prioritized before free wi-fi and the internet connectivity provision. Sri Lanka has an excellent example on this account which has some of the best social indicators from the region and where around 81% of the population resides in rural areas. Further Sri Lanka has been able to prioritize education and health in its initial planning phase which has given it an edge over other countries (in the domain of social indicators) of the region. These priorities have also contributed to building capacities to sustain in rural areas, restricting rural-urban migration.

India, which still predominately lives in villages, faces a difficult urbanization transition. India had two planned cities named Bhubaneswar and Chandigarh, conceptualized as model cities, their respective development in terms of infrastructure as well as administration is visible. Chandigarh has surpassed Bhubaneswar by a huge margin. Similarly, the cities of Faridabad and Gurugram (erstwhile known as Gurgaon) adjoin Delhi and which were initiated with allotment, allocation, and approvals around same time, however Gurugram surpassed Faridabad in almost all physical development parameters. The primary reason is their administration and the state's intervention. The experiences of these models need to be revisited and the lessons learnt from them should be more generally applied in order to make better plans for the future. Kathmandu in Nepal, Karachi in Pakistan, and Dhaka in Bangladesh, were not built for the kind of pressure they face today in terms of responding to the modern day need of the population in terms of transportation, accommodation and

---

[13]PURA is an acronym of Providing Urban Amenities in Rural Areas, given by Abdul Kalam, the former President of India. He has talked about focusing on rural prosperity and believed that it is possible by creating three connectivities—physical, electronic, and knowledge, leading to economic connectivity (see Abdul Kalam, 2012, pp. 52–53).

amenities. Satellite cities need to be developed to deal with the pressure these cities are facing. The governments of all South Asian countries must design cities to cater to future needs.

Physical infrastructure is an important impediment but what is more challenging is to revive better community living across geographies. The race for better material living has left rural areas with poor thinking on community living and sense of togetherness. The fall in human values is considered to be the major cause of social problems today. It is caused by concentration on acquiring more wealth and material goods. It needs to be examined through the provision of better primary education, teaching young children of the rich heritage of the region. Such education could help them develop a sense of pride and build better perception towards life and priorities. Efforts are required to be put to rebuild their value system, teaching them to respect all faiths and learn good virtues.

Altruistically helping others in times of need has to be nurtured in youth by sharing the success stories of great people. The role of teachers in this regard is very important as they play a pivotal role in shaping the future. Children must be surrounded by people with whom they can better connect and who can become their role models. In this environment, the role of parents, elders, and teachers is of great importance as it is not just through teaching that our future generation is going to be affected, but also through observing role models.

Cities that provide better amenities and accessibility have to also ensure better governance through citizen friendly regulations. This is major learning from the development story of Gurugram and Faridabad or Bhubaneswar and Chandigarh in India. The role of the state should be minimized to the role of watchdogs and regulators. Political leaders must set examples through their unbiased work towards more effective governance. Different states in India are developing new cities, keeping in mind future infrastructure and expansion. Livable cities need to be transformed into happy cities assuring across region for better HWB.

5.7   On Governance

Poor governance is one of the difficult challenges facing South Asia. Much of the region practices democracy but being a follower of a democratic system does not guarantee good governance. The democratic system as such is not devoid of the concentration of wealth into the hands of the few. Bose and Jalal (2004) categorically mention that the overemphasis on the consumer goods sector (especially textiles) by Pakistan influenced the country to be part of the international capitalist system deeply affecting Pakistan's future policy to be more dependent on external finances, which resulted in the concentration of wealth into the hands of the privileged. This further affected the neglect of the social sector as a whole by political leaders and successive authoritarian regimes. Bose and Jalal further state that:

It is true that India's social indicators are not appreciably better than Pakistan's. But this has less to do with the formally democratic or overtly authoritarian character of the regimes that have governed the two countries than with the state–society nexus as a whole. If there is a lesson to be learnt from India's post-colonial experience it is that the paraphernalia of democracy is a necessary but by no means sufficient condition for achieving the goal of development with social justice. (Bose & Jalal, 2004, p.192)

Talbot (1998, p. 368) stated: "There are three A's which define Pakistan's politics, they are – the Allah, the Army and the America … but if it wishes to have stability it should focus on five C's, which are – consensus, consent, commitment, conviction and compassion" (Talbot, 1998, p. 373). Deaton (2017) states that in low-income countries, governments generally seem to favor policies that increase inequality.

A study conducted by Krieger and Meierrieks (2016) on the panel data from 100 countries (including Bangladesh, India, Nepal, Pakistan, and Sri Lanka from the South Asian region) provides some hard truths. The negative impact of inequality on measures of economic freedom leads towards the use of economic power for political gain by wealthy people. These people advance their social and economic interests which is true for both democratic and non-democratic countries. It means that being a democratic country, one cannot be sure that wealthy people would not influence the policy.

While all the countries of South Asia have democratic governments, all of their governance is not truly democratic. It is a disturbing paradox that the more vigorous the South Asian democracy is, the more dysfunctional it becomes (Nepali, 2009, p. 7). There is a reminder for all these governments of what one of the founding fathers of the United States, Thomas Jefferson, said in 1809: "The care of human life and happiness, and not their destruction, is the first and only object of good government." Noah (2012) narrates the inequality present in America and Europe and its origin, finding that wherever public policies are driven by wealthy politicians catering to rich electorates, it amounts to the government not being democratic. Although this work is based on American and European experiences, it helps one understand the implications of political decisions irrespective of geographic location. This makes more sense when looking at the public policy discourse in India, Pakistan, Bangladesh, and Bhutan. It is in this light that governance as such has been much of a challenge in the region.

5.8 On Use of Technology

Technology advancements have been catalysts for change. Not just for businesses, but for the state as well. The governments of South Asia have started using technology to devise policies and to deliver them efficiently to the end users, aka the public. Digital disruption is one such initiative and Digital India is one such mission that aims to provide seamless services in an open environment assuring transparency, security, and speed. Public policy is an area which needs to embrace technology to strategize and develop appropriate policies to improve the quality of life of people and their well-being.

For the state to visualize better growth and development, two approaches are available. The first approach is to push the policies whereby driving people to learn and develop an attitude of adapting to change. Thus, it pushes the people to change without much choice. Some view it as an imposition whereas others consider it to be a necessity. Whatever the case, it is broadly considered as an approach that may lead to a better tomorrow. The second approach is to empower citizens by providing quality education so that they can make better choices and make wise decisions. Enlightening citizens through knowledge also focuses on building better social infrastructure in order to assure a better future in the long run. In this approach the citizens feel liberated and are driven to undertake initiatives, to develop the state, and to contribute positively for the prosperity of the people. The first approach gives short-term results whereas the second approach provides long-term returns.

As a state, one has to have a mix of these two approaches so that balanced growth takes place taking care of political compulsions and aspirations. Information and Communication Technology (ICT) has played a key role in empowering citizens whereby committing resources for improving HWB. Digital divide has been improved and converted into digital dividend and resulted in driving digital disruption to leverage excellent new technologies to connect with the stakeholders in a more efficient manner. The use of technology is certainly heading towards building a rich knowledgeable society and as stipulated would help HWB through digital empowerment.

Bhutan has successfully used e-governance platforms to develop and effectively deliver services to its citizens. This small, yet, important nation which follows a development philosophy termed GNH has shown its commitment to the cause of HWB. It has responded to it with appropriate initiatives using technology and digitalization for assuring transparency at all levels. The adoption of technology in Bangladesh, Bhutan, India, the Maldives, and Sri Lanka is remarkable and has improved substantially.

Digital distraction has to be handled with care and digital wellness has to be assured. Overdose of provisioning digital platforms, where education standards are low, would be a much greater challenge for all the people involved in designing and delivering digital products and services. Over use of internet by children needs to be taken care so that such a move does not negatively affect the basic social fabric of a nation. Execution and effective implementation need to be strengthened, which would only be possible when digital literacy reaches to the nooks and corners of the region.

Nations have to commit to improving the quality of their people and to looking beyond economic measures. The use of technology should be directed towards providing better and faster solutions, which would help citizens to build trust in their elected governments. Technology can be used for seamless services guaranteeing equity and indiscrimination, as human intervention could be minimized in this kind of ecosystem.

5.9 Conclusion and the Way Forward

Sri Lanka, Pakistan, Bhutan, the Maldives, and India have already reached middle-income status. Bangladesh, Nepal, and Afghanistan are lagging behind and must put policies in place to strengthen their income measures. Yet, as a whole the region has to prioritize improving the quality of life of its residents through effective policy measures leading towards improved educational achievements. An integrated South Asian region can achieve that in a more concerted way but that is a challenge in itself, looking at the kind of relationships India, Pakistan, Nepal, and Bangladesh have. Nepal and Bhutan are landlocked nations who trade primarily with India. The EU is much more interconnected to the South Asian region as compared to the United States. Though India and Pakistan share their borders, very little trade takes place between these two countries (Bhattarai, 2011, p. 262). The trade relationship between India and Pakistan needs to be improved. Positive politics through trade and commerce can strengthen ties; sports and entertainment are other areas where much more needs to be done to bring the countries together. The governments on both sides have been putting this on their agenda but breakthroughs have not been achieved.

Efforts have been made to index South Asia in terms of its transitions concerning HWB. The world has become a better place to live in as far as physical infrastructure is concerned, though this is relative. Policies are designed to satisfy the needs of the citizens so that their living standards are improved and the outcome of policies is measured in terms of targets and their achievement. Such policies may improve HWB indicators, yet whether it would improve the happiness of the people or not is unclear. That is where happiness and HWB differ. HWB is more indicator-driven whereas happiness is at cognitive level which also concerns affect. The indicators that are studied in this book attempt to compare and contrast the outcome of different domains and try communicating with the reader their respective state. The problems affecting different countries in the region are affecting their policy-making process. As mentioned previously in this monograph, between the policy formulation and execution is the delivery machinery, which is governance. For the entirety of the region (with a few minor exceptions) this delivery has been the key issue.

The major strengths, weaknesses, opportunities, and threats have been identified through previous chapters and are shown in Table 5.1 highlighting major areas of concern for different countries. Poor governance is one of the most common challenges all the countries in the region face. World over, governance has been an important issue in assuring HWB. Wherever governance is good, citizens express satisfaction and their perception is positive. Bhutan is an example of that, all its parameters are not at the top, yet when it measures well on governance, much of the things are taken care of. India, Pakistan, Bangladesh, and Sri Lanka have had around 70 years of planned development but yet the legacy with which they are burdened still shadows thinking.

Table 5.1 Regional SWOT

Country	Strengths	Weaknesses	Opportunities	Threats
Afghanistan	Strong financial and military ties with the US, land resource, oil fields, health expenditure	Lowest on most of the indicators (income, health, education, and governance), poverty	Improving health and education and providing good governance	Military, terrorism, insecurity, border relations with Pakistan
Bangladesh	Health, steady growth, low labor cost	Literacy, unemployment	Improving health and education, creation of job opportunities	Political disturbances, governance, border relations
Bhutan	Peaceful, strong relations with India, GNH as philosophy, steady economic growth, governance, size, health expenditure	Landlocked, has major trade with India, not member of WTO, education, unemployment	Improving education and health, encouraging entrepreneurship	Environment protection, border relations
India	Economic growth, health, financial resources	Population density, education, employability	Improving governance, quality of education	Governance, cross border terrorism, border relations with Pakistan and Bangladesh
The Maldives	Size of the country, income, health, literacy	Governance, environment protection, unemployment	Improving governance, protecting environment	Political instability, corruption, environment (CO_2 emission)
Nepal	Availability of doctors, steady growth	Landlocked, has major trade with India, poverty	Improving health and education	Terrorism, power struggle
Pakistan	Steady growth, close relations with China	Health, governance, poverty	Improving governance, education and health	Border relations with India and Afghanistan cross border terrorism
Sri Lanka	Population density, health, education	Governance, unemployment	Improving governance, encouraging entrepreneurship	Terrorism, sectarianism, corruption

Yet so long as managers of post-colonial states remain trapped in the colonial mould, valuable resources get frittered away in high defence expenditure occasioned by inter-state hostilities, the potential benefits of a common South Asian market remain unrealized and the promise of social and economic freedom that was supposed to follow on the heels of political independence in 1947 remains a mirage for the majority of the subcontinent's poor and obscure. (Bose & Jalal, 2004, p. 200)

It shall not continue long. Overall conditions have begun to improve and it is believed that it will further improve at a good pace. The major challenge is in improving the quality of education, which will naturally improve all other parameters. It is education and nothing else that liberates and teaches brotherhood, respect, cooperation, togetherness, and tolerance. An educational system has to have these values in order to serve their respective countries and the world.

In 2006 during the 86th session of the National Assembly and after taking office as king, Jigme Khesar Namgyel Wangchuk, commanded: "The people's welfare, at all times and in all respects, is the sacred duty of the King." (Kinga, 2009, p. 300). This statement calls for all the leaders to commit themselves to the well-being of their citizens. Leadership at different levels has to have this mindset which works to build trust with the public, and that is how the good governance can be assured to the people. Governance in education and health is primarily the foundation on which the future of a nation rests. If South Asia is able to unite and make a concerted effort it has the potential of becoming a dominant force in future.

References

Abdul Kalam, A. P. J. (2012). *Turning points—A journey through challenges.* New Delhi: Harper Collins Publishers India.

Bhattarai, K. (2011). Trade, growth and poverty in South Asia. In R. Jha (Ed.), *Routledge handbook of South Asian economics* (pp. 258–276). New York: Routledge.

Blanchflower, D. G., & Oswald, A. J. (2004). Well-being over time in Britain and the USA. *Journal of Public Economics, 88*(7–8), 1359–1386.

Bok, D. (2010). *The politics of happiness—What government can learn from the new research on well-being.* Princeton: Princeton University Press.

Bose, S., & Jalal, A. (2004). *Modern South Asia—History, culture, political economy* (2nd ed.). London: Routledge.

Carus, P. (1995). *The gospel of Buddha.* Chicago and London: The Open Court Publishing Company. Accessed from https://oll.libertyfund.org/titles/buddha-the-gospel-of-buddha.

Cobb, C., Gary, S., Goodman, & Mathis, W. (1999). Why bigger isn't better: The genuine progress indicator—1999. Update. *Redefining Progress* (November). Accessed from http://www.nber.org/rosenbla/econ302/lecture/GPIGDP/gpi1999.pdf.

Costanza, R., Hart, M., Posner, S., & Talbert, J. (2009). *Beyond GDP: The need for new measures of progress.* The Pardee Papers No. 4, January 2009. The Frederick S. Pardee Center for the Study of the Longer-Range Future. Boston University. Accessed form http://pdxscholar.library.pdx.edu/cgi/viewcontent.cgi?article=1010&context=iss_pub.

Coyle, D. (2014). *GDP—A brief but affectionate history.* Princeton: Princeton University Press.

Deaton, A. (2017). Without governments, would countries have more inequality, or less? *The Economist.* Accessed from https://www.economist.com/news/world-if/21724910-angus-deaton-nobel-prizewinning-economist-explores-question-intrigued-him-without on September 29, 2017.

Diener, E., & Seligman, M. (2004). Beyond money, towards an economy of well-being. *Psychological Science in the Public Interest, 5*(1), 1–31.

Easterbrook, G. (2003). *The progress paradox how life gets better while people feel worse.* New York: Random House.

Easterlin, R. A. (1974). Does economic growth improve the human lot? Some empirical evidence. In P. A. David & M. W. Reder (Eds.), *Nations and households in economic growth: Essays in honor of Moses Abramowitz* (pp. 89–125). NY: Academic Press.

Easterlin, R. A. (1995). Will raising the incomes of all increase the happiness of all? *Journal of Economic Behavior & Organization, 27*(1), 35–48.

Easterlin, R. A. (2001). Income and happiness: Towards a unified theory. *The Economic Journal, 111,* 465–484.

Estes, R. J., & Zhou, H. (2014). A conceptual approach to the creation of public–private partnerships in social welfare. *International Journal of Social Welfare, 24*(4). https://doi.org/10.1111/ijsw.12142.

Frey, B. S., & Stutzer, A. (2002). What can economists learn from happiness research? *Journal of Economic Literature, 40*(2), 402–435.

Goossens, Y., Makipaa, A., Philipp, S., & van de Sand, I. (2007). *Alternative progress indicators to gross domestic product (GDP) as a means towards sustainable development.* Policy Department, Economic and Scientific Policy. European Parliament. Accessed from http://www.europarl.europa.eu/RegData/etudes/etudes/join/2007/385672/IPOL-ENVI_ET(2007)385672_EN.pdf.

Helliwell, J. (2003). How's life? Combining individual and national variations to explain subjective wellbeing. *Economic Modelling, 20,* 331–360. Accessed from http://faculty.arts.ubc.ca/jhelliwell/papers/Helliwell-EM2003.pdf.

ILO. (2018). *World employment social outlook—Trends 2018.* Geneva, Switzerland: International Labor Organization.

Jackson, T. (2006). *Beyond the well-being paradox: Well-being, consumption growth, and sustainability.* CES working paper 06/06. Guildford (Surrey) UK: Centre for Environmental Strategy, University of Surrey. Accessed from https://www.surrey.ac.uk/ces/files/pdf/0606_WP_Wellbeing_and_SD.pdf.

Jackson, T. (2009). *Prosperity with growth—Economics for a finite planet.* London: Earthscan Publications.

Jebb, A. T., Tay, L., Diener, E., & Oishi, S. (2018). Happiness income satiation and turning points around the world. *Nature Human Behaviour, 2*(33–38). Accessed from https://www.nature.com/articles/s41562-017-0277-0.

Kinga, S. (2009). *Kingship and democracy—A biography of the Bhutanese state.* Thimphu: Ministry of Education, Royal Government of Bhutan.

Krieger, T., & Meierrieks, D. (2016). Political capitalism: The interaction between income inequality, economic freedom and democracy. *European Journal of Political Economy, 45,* 115–132.

Kuznets, S. (1934). *National income, 1929–32, 1934.* New York: National Bureau of Economic Research. Accessed from http://www.nber.org/chapters/c2258.pdf.

Layard, R. (2006). *Happiness: Lessons from a new science.* London: Penguin.

Maddison, A. (1995). *Monitoring the world economy 1820–1992.* Paris: OECD Development Centre.

Mathur, K. (2013). *Public policy and politics in India—How institutions matter.* New Delhi: Oxford University Press.

MaxNeef, M. (1995). Economic growth and quality of life: A threshold hypothesis. *Ecological Economics, 15*(2), 115–118.

Montgomery, C. (2013). *Happy city: Transforming our lives through urban design.* New York: Farrar, Straus and Giroux.

Nepali, R. K. (2009). *Democracy in South Asia.* Stockholm, Sweden: International Institute for Democracy and Electoral Assistance.

Noah, T. (2012). *The great divergence: America's growing inequality crisis and what we can do about it.* New York: Bloomsbury Press.

Nordhaus, W., & Tobin, J. (1973). Is growth absolute. In M. Moss (Ed.), *The measurement of economic and social performance* (pp. 509–564). NBER. Accessed from https://econpapers.repec.org/bookchap/nbrnberch/3621.htm.

Ostry, J. D., Berg, A., & Tsangarides, C. G. (2014). *Redistribution, inequality, and growth.* IMF Staff Discussion Note, February 2014. Accessed from https://www.imf.org/external/pubs/ft/sdn/2014/sdn1402.pdf.

Oxfam. (2014). *Working for the few: Political capture and economic inequality.* Oxford Briefing Paper 178. Accessed from https://www.oxfam.org/sites/www.oxfam.org/files/bp-working-for-few-politicalcapture-economic-inequality-200114-summ-en.pdf on October 20, 2017.

Piketty, T. (2014). *Capital in the 21st century.* Cambridge, MA: Harvard University Press.

Planning Commission. (2000). *Bhutan national human development report 2000—Gross national happiness and human development: Searching for common ground.* Thimphu: Planning Commission Secretariat, Royal Government of Bhutan. Accessed from http://hdr.undp.org/sites/default/files/bhutan_2000_en.pdf on January 10, 2016.

Posner, S., & Costanza, R. (2011). A summary of ISEW and GPI studies at multiple score and new estimates for Baltimore City, Baltimore Country and the state of Maryland. *Ecological Economics, 70*(11), 1972–1980.

Sen, A. (1976). Real national income. *Review of Economic Studies, 43*(1), 19–39.

Sen, A. (1979). The welfare basis of real income comparisons. *Journal of Economic Literature, 17*(1), 1–45.

Sgroi, D., Hills, T., O'Donnell, G., Oswald, A., & Proto, E. (2017). In K. Brandon (Ed.), *Understanding happiness—A CAGE policy report.* London: Centre for Competitive Advantage in the Global Economy, Social Market Foundation. Accessed from https://www.andrewoswald.com/docs/HappinessReport2017V1.pdf.

Shrotryia, V. K. (2017). The history of well-being in South Asia. In R. J. Estes & M. J. Sirgy (Eds.), *The pursuit of human well-being—The untold global history* (pp. 349–380). International Handbooks on Quality of Life. Switzerland: Springer International Publishing.

Smith, A. (1984). *The theory of moral sentiments.* Indianapolis: Liberty Fund Inc.

Stiglitz, J., Sen, A., & Fitoussi, J. (2010). *Mismeasuring our lives, why GDP does not add up.* New Delhi: Book well Publications.

Talbot, I. (1998). *Pakistan—A modern history.* London: Hurst & Company.

van den Bergh, J. C. J. M. (2007). *Abolishing GDP.* Tinbergen Institute Discussion Paper TI 2007-019/3. Accessed from https://papers.tinbergen.nl/07019.pdf.

van den Bergh, J. C. J. M. (2009). GDP paradox. *Journal of Economic Psychology, 30*(2), 117–135. https://doi.org/10.1016/j.joep.2008.12.001.

Von, T. A. (2007). *Indian summer: The secret history of the end of an empire.* London: Simon & Schuster.

Weitzman, M. (1976). On the welfare significance of the national product in a dynamic economy. *Quarterly Journal of Economics, 90,* 156–162.

Wilkinson, R., & Pickett, K. (2009). *The spirit level: Why greater equality makes societies stronger.* New York: Bloomsbury.

World Bank. (2008). *The growth report: Strategies for sustained growth and inclusive development.* Washington, DC: Commission on Growth and Development, World Bank.

World Bank. (2019). *World development report 2019: The changing nature of work.* Washington, DC: The World Bank.

Index

© Springer Nature Switzerland AG 2020
V. K. Shrotryia, *Human Well-Being and Policy in South Asia*, Human Well-Being
Research and Policy Making, https://doi.org/10.1007/978-3-030-33270-9